HONORING LOSS
GROWING THROUGH GRIEF

To request permission, contact the publisher at:
publisher@innerpeacepress.com

ISBN: 978-1-958150-25-2
Honoring Loss, Growing through Grief:
Yoga for Personal Transformation and Resilience in
Times of Transition and Loss

Subjects
SELF-HELP / Death, Grief, Bereavement
HEALTH & FITNESS / Yoga
BODY, MIND & SPIRIT / Inspiration & Personal Growth

Published by **Inner Peace Press**
Eau Claire, Wisconsin, USA
www.innerpeacepress.com

HONORING LOSS
GROWING THROUGH GRIEF

Yoga for Personal Transformation
and Resilience in Times of
Transition and Loss

MOYA MCGINN MATHEWS

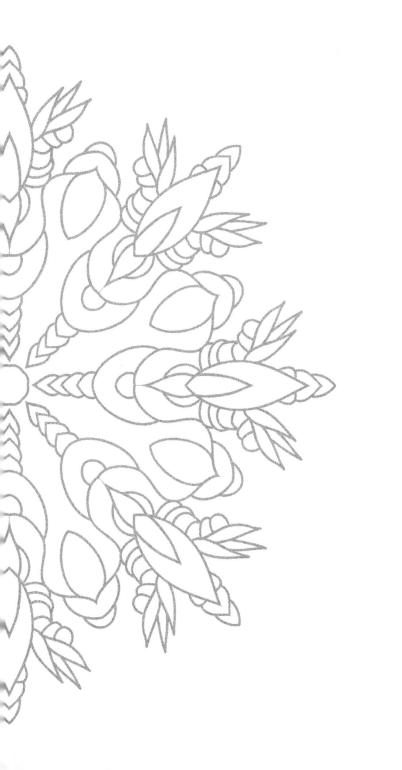

to my parents,
my first teachers,
and to all my teachers

Table of Contents

ACKNOWLEDGMENTS

"No duty is more urgent than
that of returning thanks."
~ **St. Ambrose**

In my own journey of grief, transition, loss, healing, and personal growth, there have been numerous teachers, students, counselors, and friends who have come into my life to support and guide me. My heart is thankful for all of them. This book is but one manifestation of their reminder to listen with my heart and to speak with love and wisdom. I am truly grateful.

Two prominent individuals have not only played significant roles in my personal growth and healing, they have provided steadfast support as I persevere in life and work in general, and toward the completion of this book in particular. In their great love for me, they have believed in me, in the purpose of my work, and in the concept of the book since I first dreamt of it.

My sister, Sheila, my *Anam Cara*, or "soul-friend" since my birth, has proofread and edited multiple drafts of this text. Since we were children, her unique and brilliant perspective inspired me to live with a sense of purpose, to do better work, and to be a better human, core values that were surely instilled in us by our amazing parents. I'm so grateful for Sheila, now the last living member of our family of origin, and for our bond of kinship and friendship.

My husband, Mike, my true love and soul-companion, has been a daily, constant voice of encouragement to me in every endeavor for more than two decades. His complete confidence in me has been life-changing, and he has served me coffee and cheered on my writing efforts since the first paragraphs of this book were composed at our kitchen table. Mike is the one who unfailingly has my back, both figuratively and literally, as you will see in a few of the photos in which he makes a cameo appearance. Other than those photos that include him, he was the photographer for all of the images. Also, he makes me laugh, and I do not under-estimate the healing power of that laughter.

Comforted by the words of the great Meister Eckhart, "If the only prayer you said was thank you, that would be enough," I do indeed say, "Thank you," and hope it is enough.

Moya McGinn Mathews
Minneapolis, MN
October 2023

FOREWORD

Moya McGinn Mathews has distilled the knowledge and sensibilities of 40 years of pastoral ministry and 20 years of yoga into this inviting and accessible handbook for using yoga to engage with and move beyond grief. Mathews critiques the mere pious platitudes often heard about "getting over" grief. She provides the heartfelt reasons why those perspectives are woefully inadequate and provides an alternative mind-and-body practice to work through grief and its aftershocks. Nor is yoga here presented as a purely mechanical set of "fitness" tools. Mathews introduces the ancient science underlying various yogic poses and practices, explaining why such poses affect the mind-and-body in specific ways. This "workbook" takes both grief and yoga seriously, presenting both in an eminently readable and personal way for grief survivors on the path to wholeness.

Early in the volume, the author's brief reprise of the series of losses she has endured makes the case for her credibility in dealing with grief. But those who themselves have experienced grief will realized that the brief list of losses barely scratches the surface of the experiences themselves. As her niece commented after the sudden death of the author's husband, "Moya's life sucks." Truly, we know that grief sucks, both in the colloquial sense of the expression and also in the emotional and physiological senses. Living in grief can become a physical and emotional black hole. But it need not be so. This handbook provides guidance for using yoga to work in, with, and through grief so it does not become that area of your life with a gravitational pull so strong that nothing has sufficient energy to escape it.

I have had the great privilege of watching this book progress from its inception to this, its final form. This volume represents the author's journey through grief, in which I've had the heartbreaking privilege to participate. I'm so proud of Moya for what she has achieved in this volume, and for the gift she provides to her readers who are struggling with that "black hole" experience of grief and loss. There is hope. There is light. *Honoring Loss, Growing through Grief* provides a beacon for all of us who walk daily in the shadows of loss and grief.

Sheila E. McGinn, PhD
Emerita Professor of Theology & Religious Studies
John Carroll University
Cleveland, Ohio

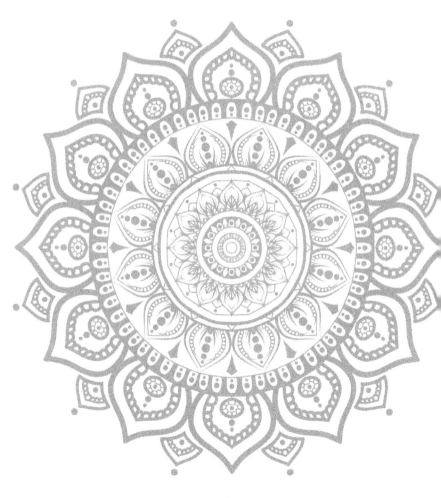

Introduction

I recently attended an interview for a yoga teaching job. The interviewer asked, "What's the most difficult challenge that you've ever faced?" I didn't have to deliberate long and hard. If I delayed in answering, it was because I thought my answer was too personal for a professional conversation. "When I was 38 years old, my husband suddenly dropped dead," I responded.

More than two decades after that fateful day, Chad's death remains to be the challenging life transition against which I measure all other challenges, thinking, "I navigated that profound and painful loss, and I can get through this current situation." In the weeks immediately prior to that interview, I had suffered professional losses. I was being abused by my boss at my primary place of employment, my position and salary had been cut by more than 15%, and I was continuing to endure a very hostile work environment. As difficult as it was for me to hold myself together through that horrible and painful situation, I knew I would get through it, outlast it, and rise above it because I had been through far worse personal and emotional turmoil.

I would not be the person I am today had I not experienced grief and loss, and I am truly grateful for who I am and for all that I am becoming. Courage, faith, resilience, integrity, and empathy are just a few of the personal qualities I've discovered within myself. These qualities are part of my core. Other personal qualities which I value, like patience and the serenity of surrender, don't seem to come as naturally to me, so I intentionally work to cultivate them, and I live into the paradox that true surrender requires real faith and courage.

Please know this: whatever you're going through, you can do this. I won't suggest that you'll ever "get over," this thing called grief, but you can get through it. My recent job-related suffering has reminded me that grief follows a cyclical pattern, and new challenges, transitions, and hurts can trigger old wounds. But I have learned that I am greater than my wounds.

You are also greater than your wounds. You may be in pain and suffering right now, but pain and suffering need not be the end of the story. Grieving is a process of healing, and needs time, patience, rest, nourishment, and support.

I haven't done any of this alone, and you don't have to, either. I've been sustained by a Power far greater than my own, and surrounded by supportive allies on the healing journey – family, friends, and simpatico companions. Geese fly faster and farther when they travel in a flock. Humans thrive when we bond in healthy and purposeful communities. When you are ready, find an individual or group to support your process.

The parable of falling into a hole

A story is told of a woman cheerfully walking down the street. Suddenly and unexpectedly she falls into a hole. The hole is dark and bleak. It is so deep and its walls so steep, she can't climb out. Filled with anguish and despair, she cries out for help.

A psychiatrist walks past, hears her plea for assistance, and writes her a prescription. "Here," says the doctor, dropping the prescription down into the hole. "Take these pills; they should ease the pain." The doctor walks on. Still stuck in her predicament, the trapped woman continues to wail aloud.

A monk walks past. "I'll pray for you," he says sincerely. While the thought of his prayers momentarily soothes the woman's soul, she realizes that she is still stuck down in the hole, alone, anxious, and afraid. Others pass by and observe the woman's plight. They give her offerings of self-help books, coffee gift cards, and bus tokens. As generous as their contributions, nothing changes the reality that she is stuck in a hole.

Finally a friend walks past the hole and hears her lamentations. Immediately, her friend jumps into the hole with her. "Great," the woman exclaims. "Now we're both stuck in this hole." Her friend answers, "Yes, but I've been down in this hole before, and I know a way out."

Dear reader, I've been down in the hole of grief, and I know a way out.

Why Yoga for Grief, Transition, and Loss?

In the months that followed the death of my husband in April of 2000, as I conversed with close friends about my experience and my reflections on death and life, grief and loss, they would often say to me, "You should write a book." I actually agreed with them. I thought that I would certainly write a book about my experience of grief and transition in the hopes that my voice would comfort and support another person working through a similar process.

A few years passed and I came up with plenty of reasons *not* to write a book. I didn't have time; I was too busy raising a child, earning a living, caring for an aging parent. The routine duties of daily life and the "tyranny of the urgent" pulled me away from the desire and drive to write about my experience. Self-doubt crept in; maybe I lacked the discipline and focus required to compose a book. I dropped the idea long enough to argue that I was "too far away" from the experience of being widowed to speak to it in an authentic way. The moment had passed. I'm remarried, I'm happy. I've "moved forward."

What I really needed was a good reason to write. I needed to sense that I had something to offer that was unique, and relatively unexplored or under-developed by other contributors to the body of material available for the grieving.

In 2006 I completed my first yoga teacher training and began teaching yoga. Over the course of several years, I started offering yoga workshops for grief, transition, and loss. When I first began researching and preparing to teach these workshops, I realized that there really wasn't much "out there" on the topic of yoga for grief. I saw that I did have something unique to contribute, and this practice of **Yoga for Grief, Transition, and Loss** was conceived.

I've been down in the hole of grief, and have seen that yoga can provide a way out.

I survived grief, and you can too. Please know that you will survive. You may even thrive, though not necessarily immediately. Be patient with the process.

This book offers useful yogic tools for this process. It is offered for persons navigating grief, and can be used at any stage of the process, even long after the wake of traumatic grief seems to have subsided. The reality is that life is always in transition, so these tools are for a lifetime.

Exercises offered in this book include deep, yogic breathing, yoga postures linked with breathing patterns, meditation, visualization, and journaling exercises for self-reflection. The book can be used by an individual as a guide for a yoga home practice and self-study, or can be used by a grief support group under the guidance of a yoga teacher or counselor. The process of grief is uniquely personal for every individual. Yoga as a therapeutic practice lends itself readily to personalization, adaptation, and modification. While a yoga practice will be deeply personal for each practitioner, sharing the experience with a circle of supportive companions enhances the healing process, helping us experience in a concrete way that we are not alone.

What is Yoga?

Yoga is sometimes translated as "integration" or "union." The practice of yoga leads us toward union with our most authentic Self and union with the Source of our being.

The word "yoga" comes from a Sanskrit word meaning "to join" or "to yoke" – the kind of yoke one might use to join horses or oxen to a cart, chariot, or other vehicle of transportation. In yoga, we yoke our personal story, experience, and practice to the wisdom of the sages, prophets, and teachers – past and present – to help us live authentically as we journey forward in life.

Yoga evolved from experiments and discoveries of the sages of ancient India who worked with various practices such as ethical conduct, physical postures, breathing, meditation, and concentration. In their exploration, the sages developed profoundly beneficial methods which have been passed forward by yoga teachers for thousands of years.

Modern medicine, psychology, and other sciences are now not only verifying the healing possibilities that a well-constructed yoga practice can offer; they are also contributing to the diverse ways that yoga is developing today. As doctors, healers, yoga teachers, and practitioners integrate the wisdom of modern science with these ancient yogic practices, yoga's evolution continues. We owe tremendous gratitude to the sages and teachers of India for developing the practice of yoga. It's important to note that no single culture, nation, or religious sect "owns" yoga. The notion that it originally or definitively belongs to a single, particular religious sect ignores yoga's rich historical diversity. The practice of yoga is not concerned with any one deity, Godhead, or religious sect or tradition. Any person of any religious tradition, or no religious persuasion, can practice yoga.

What is yoga practice?

Yoga practice is as elemental as 1) breathing, 2) moving, and 3) focusing the mind enough to consciously link breath and movement. Any person capable of these three activities can practice yoga. In yoga practice, the conscious linking of breath and movement, or breath and stillness, is used to cultivate mindfulness and awareness in the present moment.

What is Grief?

What if I told you that I know of a process that offers the opportunity for tremendous personal growth and learning? The benefits of this process could include:

- » discerning a new sense of your life's purpose
- » finding a more intimate connection to other people and to your true Self
- » growing in compassion and gaining new perspective and insights
- » developing a deeper sense of strength, confidence, courage, and hope

This all sounds pretty exciting, doesn't it? Maybe you're thinking, "Sign me up!" There's just one hitch: you really don't sign up. This process is called grief.

Just as there is no "one size fits all" yoga, there is no one, universal experience of grief. Grief is universally human in the sense that everyone will experience grief at some point in life, but no two people will experience it in identical ways.

Grief can feel like a pit in the stomach, tension in the chest, or pain in the heart; grief can manifest as the exhausting inability to sleep or the lack of desire to get out of bed, the inability to stop crying or the inability to shed a single tear. Grief may bring feelings of regret, fear, denial, anger, remorse, anxiety, and depression. Grief can disrupt our sense of self and identity and can make us feel lost, helpless, and afraid.

Grief is not the linear experience as we might infer from clinical theories such as the five stages or seven stages of grief. Grief is a graduated process, but there is no "graduation from" grief. Grief is more like a labyrinth with cycles, spirals, and loops. Often, just when we think we're "over" something or we've "dealt with" it, old emotional wounds may be triggered. We may be challenged to face and heal these wounds anew at a more profound level.

While grief brings challenge and turmoil, grief can also bring tremendous personal growth and learning. Grief can be the catalyst to lead us to introspection and self-reflective practices, resulting in greater clarity in many areas of life. We may find a renewed sense of direction and purpose. We may develop a more intimate connection to our deepest, truest Self and become clearer and more intentional in our relationships with others. Having experienced grief, we may grow in compassion, empathy, perspective, and insight.

Grief can help us become more deeply aware of our own strength and resilience. We may grow in confidence and courage. We may learn how to ask for and receive help from others. We may connect with a deeper sense of faith and hope within ourselves. The transformative power of grief is available to those who choose to enter into the process of grieving with an open mind and heart. When we move through the process of grief, we emerge renewed. The only way out is through, and there is no turning back – no going back to *"the way things were before."*

Grief is part of being human. We're all going to die and everyone we love is going to die. Grief will touch us all, and there is no universal manual for the grieving process. This book does not presume to be a grief manual. Rather, it is a guidebook for yogic practices, techniques for practitioners to work in a safe space with a spirit of self-acceptance, creating daily, mindful practices that include self-examination and reflection, *pranayama* (breathing), *asana* (postures), conscious relaxation, and meditation. The practices are designed to allow the energy of life experiences, particularly those that we find difficult, uncomfortable, stressful, and emotionally painful, to flow through us so we can be free to accept the healing that is available to us, fully embrace the goodness of life as it is, and awaken to a new life, a new way of being.

Journal Entry: Grief is ....

(This journaling exercise can be repeated many times. Date each entry.)

WHAT IS LOSS?

I am personally cautious about the use of the word "loss" as compared to the word "death." After my mother died, I didn't say, "I lost my mom." I said, "My mom died." In the early months, that statement was usually followed by a small choke and some tears. But when people said to me, "I'm sorry for your loss," I felt comforted and heard it as a sincere and fitting expression of sympathy. When my mom died, I felt as though I had lost so much! It was as though I had lost a part of myself, and that feeling of loss was accompanied by physical, visceral sensations of emptiness. While I believe my mom's love lives on with me forever, her real, reliable, and tangible emotional support and friendship, if not gone, seemed so far away. I had lost the part of my life on this earth which included my mom's physical presence, the sound of her voice and her laughter, the sight of her radiant smile, the embrace of her warm hugs. I lost part of my family history because my mom was the keeper of the stories. I lost the opportunity to hear those stories and write them down for future generations. I lost my role as "daughter." I wasn't fired, but I lost the job of being a daughter and I became an orphan. My mother's death was an event that dramatically changed my life and created many experiences of loss for me.

We lose lots of things without misplacing them; there is a significant difference. We lose some of life's most precious gifts, and that loss can bring intense suffering. We can lose a treasured relationship, a job, our livelihood and source of income; we can lose our health, we can even lose body parts. I have a friend who lost both breasts to cancer. She didn't "misplace" them; she LOST them. They didn't accidentally fall out of her body while she wasn't paying attention. She was diagnosed with cancer and they were surgically removed in the hopes that it would save her life. That's loss; it's different than mere misplacement or absent-minded forgetting. Her medical care team even reconstructed two new breasts for her, but her body has been through incredible trauma and she has suffered loss.

The death of my dad, my husband, my brother, and my mom felt like invasive surgery, or worse. I experienced trauma and loss. I say, "they died." I don't say, "I lost them." But the word "loss" is a way for me to acknowledge and name the reality of my own experience, and naming my experience helps me to stay sane and present and empowered to work through it. I'd never suggest that loss is a synonym or euphemism for death, but loss is an experience of those who grieve.

Life is change and change includes loss. Whether the loss of a loved one, the loss of a pet, the loss of a job, a home, health, or income, the loss of security or friends, body image or sense of self worth, the loss of a role we once played for others or the loss of a relationship – transition and loss leaves a residue of grief in our physical, energetic, and emotional body. Modern science is even hypothesizing that trauma and grief can change our DNA, that the memory of traumatic experiences can be genetically inherited from our ancestors and passed forward to future generations.

The reality of all life is that we are constantly in transition, as life ebbs and flows between loss and gain. Grief includes the ever-present knowledge that we must find ways to live with loss and not allow loss to live in place of us. Grief involves constant reflection and adjustment. As we move through the grieving process, we are presented with the opportunity to grow in adaptability.

No two people will ever grieve the same way, with the same intensity, or for the same period of time. As we move through the process of grief, it is important to understand and accept the basic truth that people grieve differently. Acknowledging that the universal human experience called "grief" is profoundly personal and unique for every individual allows us to more fully accept our own manner of grieving. We also can be more accepting of and compassionate toward others who grieve and experience loss.

This practice and process of **Yoga for Grief, Transition, and Loss** encourages the practitioner to honor, acknowledge, mourn, and move through loss, lest the energy of grief remain trapped in our bodies, keeping us from the flow of our lives and even making us ill. *Honoring Loss, Growing through Grief* begins with the practice of compassion toward ourselves. When we are truly compassionate toward ourselves we can extend that compassion toward others.

"There are days when you wake up happy;
Again inside the fullness of life,
Until the moment breaks
And you are thrown back
Onto the black tide of loss.
Days when you have your heart back,
You are able to function well
Until in the middle of work or encounter,
Suddenly with no warning,
You are ambushed by grief."
~ **John O'Donohue, from the poem "For Grief"**

Journal Entry: Loss is...

(This journaling exercise can be repeated many times. Date each entry.)

How can I support a grieving student, friend, or loved one?
Each person's experience of grief is unique, and when we're navigating significant life transitions, every day is a "new normal." Here are some tips for offering authentic support to someone who is grieving.

* **Welcome people to come as they are.**

* **Create the space for compassion to arise.** Offer real support, both physical and emotional. Creating an environment in which someone feels seen and heard can reduce stress and even chronic pain.

* **Listen compassionately.** Ask grieving people how they are doing and listen in a non-judgmental manner. Reflect on the feelings they are expressing and help them explore their feelings and the reality of the death or loss.

* **Let them 'tell their story' as many times as they need.**

* **Allow periods of silence.**

* **Allow the grieving person to make choices.**

* **Observe.** We can't assume that we know what a grieving person needs. We must ask, and allow time and space for the answer.

* **Ask yourself, "What am I able to do?"**

❀ **Respect their personal space.** If planning a personal visit, it's respectful to call ahead. If calling on the phone, it's respectful to ask, "Is this a good time for you to chat, or would you prefer to call me back?" Again, allow the grieving person to make choices.

❀ **Notice and acknowledge in a positive way the effort that a grieving person is putting into the healing process.** Share that there are NO right or wrong behavior for grieving – everyone is different.

❀ **Let the grieving person set the pace for the process, and help them know that emotional set backs are part of the grief process.**

❀ **Know that a person will always grieve a loss, though in time will learn to live with it.**

❀ **Encourage the celebration of the life of the one who has died.**

❀ **Help those who are in the process of grieving develop rituals.** Ceremony can be very helpful in managing the emotions of the early difficult times and anniversaries and milestones moving forward.

❀ **Refer when necessary.** If the person who is in grief is suicidal it is your moral and ethical responsibility to refer them to a mental health professional.

"You can pretend to care, but you can't
pretend to show up."
~ **Moya McGinn Mathews**

Work towards integration of your own experiences of grief, transition, and loss

In order to offer authentic support to someone who is grieving, we must become acquainted with and comfortable with our own experiences of loss and life transition. As essential as it is to become well-acquainted with our own experiences of grief and loss, it is also important that we not insert our experience into that of a friend or student. We cannot know exactly what someone else is experiencing. In order to respectfully hold space for someone else's grief, we need to get ourselves "out of the way."

This is why we cannot take shortcuts in processing and integrating our own experiences of loss. Much like the emergency instructions on an airplane, we must put on our own oxygen mask before assisting other travelers. When we are conscientious about doing our own personal work, then we can be free to listen and support others without insinuating ourselves into their personal story. Developing personal boundaries that are strong enough to allow us to be truly present for the sake of another requires time, patience, practice, and sacrifice.

My Personal Loss Inventory

Loss of:

- Safety
- Grandchild(ren)
- Fertility
- Faith
- Partner
- Close Relative
- Religion
- Career
- Independence
- Self-worth
- Pregnancy
- Child or children
- Mother
- Grandparent(s)
- Possessions
- Father
- Job
- Health
- Sister
- Home
- Sight
- Brother
- Safety
- Family

- Pet
- Marriage
- Friendship
- Body parts
- Hearing
- Baby
- Hair
- Youth
- Dreams
- Community
- Self-Esteem
- Self-expression
- Freedom
- Mobility
- Income
- Trust
- Family
- Relationship(s)
- Childhood
- Vocation
- Sexual Function
- Body Image
- Sense of Sexuality
- Sense of Wellbeing

Secondary Losses

The death of a loved one may set in motion a wide range of other losses. Death can have a ripple effect; it can set off many other disturbances in its wake. Perhaps you have experienced secondary losses, including the following:

- Loss of emotional support and friendship
- Loss of a primary relationship
- Loss of other dependent relationships (in-laws, friends)
- Loss of the familiar way of relating to family and friends
- Loss of family structure
- Loss of support systems
- Loss of income and financial security
- Loss of dreams for the future
- Loss of ability to make decisions
- Loss of ability to focus and function
- Loss of ability to see choices
- Loss of birth order
- Loss of a chosen lifestyle
- Loss of identity
- Loss of trust
- Loss of security
- Loss of health
- Loss of home
- Loss of the past
- Loss of a part of oneself
- Loss of faith
- Loss of a sense of humor
- Loss of patience
- Loss of self-confidence

Other losses ~ journal reflection

In the past, when I have emerged from other losses and transitions into a new life and identity, what personal strengths and resources did I employ?

How did I seek out help and support from others?

What personal character strengths allowed me to persevere, survive, and eventually thrive?

We can't always know in the midst of a transition whether an experience is positive or negative, a loss or a gain. As challenging as it may be, it can sometimes be helpful to see how life unfolds before labeling an experience as "good," or "bad," or before becoming attached to a certain explanation of its meaning. Is there an example from your life of an event which at first seemed like a loss, and later turned out to be gain or good fortune?

How did you actively participate in the process of bringing about a generative outcome from grief or a life transition that you initially experienced as misfortune?

Aha! Yoga

It's difficult for me to identify the precise and memorable moment of my personal "initiation" into the process of growth and transformation called "grief." I'm sure I experienced it already as a young child, around the age of seven, when my family moved from my beloved home in a small town in Iowa to a new city. I remember feeling sad, afraid, distressed, and anxious as I anticipated and lived through the transition. That combination of emotional and psychological experiences could rightfully have been called "grief." Looking back, I see that in my childhood I sustained other losses that created sadness and grief-like experiences:

> » my sister moved away to go to college when I was about 13
> » our family dog died not long after
> » my brother had a significant psychotic break and was diagnosed with bi-polar disorder when I was 15

» my father was diagnosed with terminal cancer and died when I was 21

» by the time I was 30, my first marriage was clearly headed for divorce, and when the marriage ended, the divorce brought intense grief and distress combined with feelings of guilt, remorse, and shame

Still, the experience of grief in my life grew exponentially more intense and memorable when, at age 38, my second husband died suddenly and I became a widow.

One sunny Thursday morning in April 2000, my husband and I said our usual goodbyes as he headed off to work. Sometime that afternoon he laid his head down on his desk and died. "Cardiomyopathy," the coroner reported. That's a long, fancy word for dead. In an instant, I became a 38-year-old widow, and the single mother of a grieving adolescent. I ached not only with my own grief, but also with the pain of feeling powerless to alleviate the suffering of my 11-year-old son. Not long after my husband's death, my 50-year-old brother died of congestive heart failure. My father had died two decades earlier of colon cancer, so I was intimately familiar with sorrow and grief, but I had forgotten how grief could leave me feeling completely un-done and disassociated from myself.

After my husband died, I distinctly remember having moments in which I thought my life was unreal; I was watching it as if on a movie screen. There are parts of the movie that

I don't remember very well. Simply being present in my own life was profoundly painful.

Rituals and ceremonies

I had worked my entire career as a professional pastoral minister of music and had helped hundreds of families plan ceremonies to honor their deceased loved ones and bring comfort to their own grieving hearts. I had valuable spiritual tools and resources, and I created the most beautiful funeral services ever for my husband and my brother. My son and I made memory books filled with photos, stories, memorabilia of lives past combined with hand written reflections and tributes. We still ached. One morning after he woke up, my son came into my room and said, "Mommy, I feel like I have a big hole in my tummy." I responded, "Me, too." And we cried. How could we authentically pass through this mystery of grief and allow it to pass through us?

Grief support and grief therapy

I did and still do value talk therapy and the practice of companioning. I have been fortunate to know good therapists and companions who could listen to my story and allow me the space to process it in my own way. As a young widow in 2000, I was blessed to be part of an excellent grief support group with men and women close to my age who had lost partners.

My adult group met simultaneously with a group for children who had lost parents, so my son had access to his own experience of grief support. Talking through our experiences with compassionate listeners helped us at a cognitive, intellectual, and emotional level. We needed authentic connection, not just sympathy. Still, as useful as grief group conversations were, they didn't address the physiological impact of grief on my body. After the sudden death of my husband, every cell of my body held the experience of trauma.

Grief, trauma, and the physical body

I am not a sedentary person by habit; after my husband died I knew intuitively that I needed to move. I took up gardening, and tore up most of my entire yard by hand, mixing peat and manure in the soil for a new landscape. As part of my landscaping "therapy," my son and I manually laid down a quarter ton of boulder with only the help of a wheel barrow. While the external landscape around our home became more abundant and fruitful, my internal landscape remained desolate.

I had been a distance runner for decades, and I logged more miles the summer of 2000 than any other period of my life. As the saying goes, "You can run, but you can't hide." Disassociation always has its price. In the summer of 2001, I found a lump on my left breast and had to have surgery. Two months after the lumpectomy, I faced near-emergency surgery to remove my gallbladder. The energy of fear, pain, suffering, and intense sadness was stuck in my bodily tissue, and the thought occurred to me that I really didn't want to just keep having my aching parts cut out in a hospital operating room. I had to find a better way to address the strong and clear message that my body was giving me. It was stressed, unhappy, hurting, and "stuck." All of my external activity was holding my internal pain somewhat at bay, but it wasn't healing me or helping me get "un-stuck" from the hole I was in.

Finding a more wholistic way

For me, yoga was and is the better, more integrated way to move through difficulty, grief, trauma, and loss. When I discovered yoga, I didn't really know what it was, but I knew I needed to do it. I remember being on my mat, standing in a warrior pose. My arms were stretched wide open. My heart was exposed and vulnerable, and I still felt stable as I stood powerfully on my own two feet. I experimented with consciously synchronizing my breath with subtle adjustments in the pose and then with a sequence of poses. I felt the pulse of my strength and vitality as I simply connected to the steady rhythm of my own breath and stretched and moved my body in every direction. I sensed the energy of my life, my own miraculous life, surging through me. Could this practice be healing and transformative? When I rested in *savasana*, the final resting pose of a yoga practice, tears ran down my cheeks. At first I returned to class often, and then every day. More than one of my yoga teachers approached me to ask, "Have you considered training to be a yoga teacher?" After a third teacher posed this question to me, I asked, "Where would I go to do that?" She directed me to the Yoga Center of Minneapolis. I didn't know that I would teach, but knew I was ready to dive into a deeper level of practice and study.

Moving through life experience and moving energy through me

Through yoga study and practice, I started to learn techniques to move energy in more subtle ways, to heal myself emotionally, energetically, and physically. The ancient healing techniques of yoga led me through the center of the pain of grief and loss so I could re-discover my own center. I learned to be still. I re-learned to flow with life, to feel and digest it, to assimilate the benefits of my experience and lay aside what was no longer useful. Knowing that no one else could do this work for me, I practiced every day.

When I really learned how to breathe, the power of the practice came alive for me and I knew I needed to share it. I practiced breathing and postures and attitudes like non-struggle, non-aggression, self-acceptance, strength, courage, power, compassion, gratitude, and an openness to grace. I opened my heart to the healing power of the community at the Yoga Center of Minneapolis where I practiced and where I was honored to become one of the senior teachers. Through practice, I continue to learn to stand in my personal power with an open heart, receptive and ready to face the unknown without fear. This, for me, is the heart of yoga.

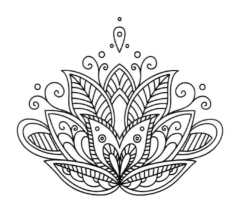

"Through yoga practice,
I continue to learn to stand
in my personal power with an open heart,
receptive and ready
to face the unknown without fear.
This, for me, is the heart of yoga."
~ **Moya McGinn Mathews**

Yoga for Self-Compassion

Yoga: yoking, joining, integrating

My immediate sense that I was experiencing something profoundly useful the very first time I witnessed the yoking of my breath with a yoga posture; it makes perfect sense to me today as I reflect back on that moment. At the time, I was still rocking in the wake of the experience of grief. Grief had left me alienated from my own body, my own life, and my own experience. Yoga brought me back to my body and back to being willing to feel my experience and my life. As I expanded the "edges" of the opening in my physical body, I noted that the "edges" of my emotional and energetic body also expanded. I found more love, more freedom, more grace, and more laughter. I was able to really laugh again!

Yoga as a science and a path

Yoga is not a religion, a cult, or a philosophy. Yoga is a science. The science of the path of *Rāja Yoga*, or Royal Yoga, is presented in the *Yoga Sutras* of Patanjali. This text is a very unique text in human history because it is not secular but it is also not related to a particular religious sect. The path of yoga as detailed by Patanjali is an eight-limbed path, including techniques to help practitioners find their own path to the light of wisdom and integration through personal experience, discipline, practice, and self-study.

Persons of any religion can combine the practice of yoga with religious practice to bring depth and richness to their faith experience. "Love your neighbor as yourself," is a biblical precept that reverberates in the heart of yoga. In yoga, we practice self-love and self-acceptance as a way of self-actualization and integration. After my husband died, one of the best pieces of advice I received was from a pastor who told me, "Be gentle with yourself." The practice of yoga helped me learn and practice gentleness and compassion towards myself.

Self-compassion practice

The age-old wisdom of self-love is being validated in contemporary times by western psychological science. Psychologists and researchers are testing the hypothesis that self-compassion as a practice is more powerful and transformational than practices of building self-esteem, and the results favor self-compassion practice. Self-compassion leads to personal improvement, because self-compassion begins from a place of self-acceptance. Research shows that when we are self-compassionate, we are more willing to make needed changes in our lives, less afraid of new challenges and experiences, more able to learn from endeavors that don't go well or as planned, and have more courage to try again. Self love is not selfish; it is essential to healthy and life-giving relationships.

Dr. Kristin Neff of the University of Texas at Austin is a pioneer in researching the effects of the practice of self-compassion. Her work demonstrates how giving ourselves a break and accepting our imperfections can be a first step toward better health. People who scored high on the self-compassion test which she designed were less depressed and anxious, and tended to be happier and more optimistic.

Self-compassion and making room for emotions

Emotions need to be heard, held, and received, not denied, coddled, fixed, or judged. Sometimes we judge emotions, whether our own or someone else's, because we don't know what else to do with them. Healing requires merciful awareness of those parts of ourselves that are in pain.

Practicing self-compassion means that we treat ourselves at least as kindly, patiently, and mercifully as we might treat our beloved child or our best friend

Begin by making a choice to try a new approach in your way of thinking about yourself. Commit to treating yourself with kindness and loving yourself unconditionally. Be gentle with yourself, let go of self-judgment, and silence the inner critic. These are all ways to describe a self-compassion practice.

Practicing compassion toward anyone, be it someone else or ourselves, requires us to first recognize that someone is suffering and then to tune into the person's experience of suffering. So the first step in the practice of self-compassion is to notice when we are suffering. This might sound very simple, but if the suffering is caused by self-judgment or self-criticism, this first step can be very challenging.

The second step in a compassion practice is to extend caring, supportive kindness in response to suffering, so in self-compassion practice, we extend authentic caring and supportive kindness to ourselves. We might do this through meditation, visualization, or practices of deep rest, relaxation, and restoration. If the inner critic is chattering, we meet that voice kindly and firmly, coaching ourselves with thoughts like "I am doing the best I can in this moment," or "all humans make mistakes," or "even though I'm feeling ____, I still deeply love and accept myself." Dr. Neff suggests various exercises such as writing yourself a letter of support, just as you might to a friend whose suffering causes you to feel concerned. She also recommends periodic "compassion breaks," placing both hands over our own heart and repeating a *mantra* (a word to support meditation) such as, "I'm going to be kind to myself in this moment."

The third step in compassion practice is to remember that suffering is part of the universal human experience;

one who suffers is not isolated. We are not alone. We might imagine linking hands with all of suffering humanity as a gesture of mutuality and support.

Finally, if we want to make the shift toward self-compassion a sustainable practice in the long run, we take notice of the difference between how we feel when we are caught up in self-criticism, as compared to how we feel when we let it go. Noticing how good it feels to practice kindness, empathy, and compassion toward ourselves and others helps us to "hack in" to a reward-based system of learning, and will motivate us to practice self-compassion more consistently.

As we practice self-compassion, we cannot neglect the very practical actions which insure that all our basic needs are met, such as healthy food and sufficient rest.

"Compassion directed to oneself is humility."
~ Simone Weil

Self-compassion reflection exercise

Think of a recent event in your life that has been unpleasant, uncomfortable, and has caused suffering for you. Close your eyes and remember the event.

※ *What do you feel?*
※ *What emotional sensations are present as you recall the event or situation?*
※ *Where do those sensations show up in your body?*

"I am" statements tend to create identification with a specific emotional experience. Your identity is so much greater than your emotional experience in this moment, your story, or your biography. As you name the feelings and emotions, try to avoid "I am" statements such as, "I am angry," or "I am frightened." These "I am" statements lead to equating an experience which is temporary with your true identity. Emotions show up in the body in feelings such as a tight throat, constriction in the chest, tension in the belly, or feeling hot or cold. To respect the sacredness of your identity, note the feelings that are present, and as you feel these sensations and note that "sensations of anger are present" or "sensations of fear are present."

- *Can you extend caring and kindness to yourself? What words of encouragement or affirmation might you say to yourself in this situation? Place both hands over your heart and gently give yourself a mini hug.*
- *Remember that all sentient beings suffer. Suffering is part of the human condition. Imagine joining hands with others who are suffering. You are not alone.*
- *How do you feel now? What emotional and physical sensations does the practice of self-compassion create?*

You may want to create a journal entry reflecting on this exercise.

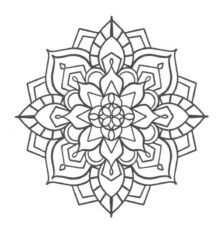

Yoga as a practice of self-compassion

Yoga uses many compassionate techniques to bring the practitioner back to wholeness, oneness, and wellness. Yoga is deeply personal; the most useful and appropriate practices and techniques for me may be very different from the techniques which are most appropriate and beneficial for you. A few very simple techniques may be enough to dramatically transform the way we experience our lives. *Ayurveda*, an ancient system of Indian medicine, is the sister science of yoga. A qualified yoga teacher or ayurvedic consultant can help a practitioner determine practices and techniques that are most appropriate and beneficial for the individual. Ultimately, your personal intuition may be the best guide to your most useful practices.

This book does not offer a "one size fits all" prescription for yoga and grieving; it offers various practices from which you can choose and design your own personal practice. The primary medium with which we will work in this practice is the practice of breathing mindfully, linking breath to postures, and intentional movement and transitions. Breath is a principal tool used in yoga to connect the body and mind and help the practitioner be awake and present in the moment.

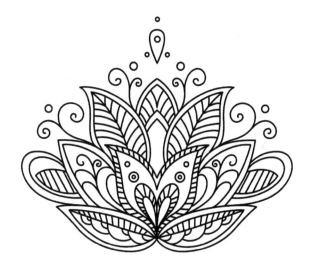

"It is not the weight you carry
but how you carry it—
books, bricks, grief—
it's all in the way
you embrace it, balance it, carry it
when you cannot, and would not,
put it down."
~ Mary Oliver

Self awareness inventory

Grief is a natural response to loss. It is often misdiagnosed as anxiety or depression, but it is its own process and it is part of being human. You may recognize in yourself some of the following emotional and behavioral patterns that can emerge in the grieving process.

Behavioral reactions

- Detached from Self, family, and friends
- Changes in interests or activities
- Change in relationships
- Change in productivity
- Changes in activity level
- Creating an extremely busy schedule to avoid feeling
- Withdrawing from regular activities and friends
- Buying things not really needed
- Isolation
- Loneliness
- Short tempered, impatient

Emotional reactions

- Feeling stunned, dazed, or overwhelmed
- Constant thoughts about the deceased person, lost job, or relationship, etc.
- Anxiety due to a change of routine
- Disbelief or denial of the reality
- Feeling vulnerable or unsafe

- Changes in mood, such as irritability, lethargy, and/or erratic mood shifts
- Intense feelings
- Feelings of abandonment
- Avoiding personal feelings
- Inability to feel or express feelings
- Panic and fear
- Sadness and numbness
- Anger, anxiety, shock, and disbelief
- Feelings of guilt or regret for things done or not done, said or not said
- Heightened sensitivity to other peoples' comments
- Easily angered
- Inclination toward argumentative behavior

Cognitive reactions
- Worries about the health and safety of self or others
- Difficulty concentrating
- Difficulty with decision making
- Preoccupation with the loss
- Need to repeat the details of the loss
- Distracted
- Decreased attention span
- Short-term memory loss
- Confusion
- Lowered self-esteem
- Believing no one understands

Physical reactions

- ⚡ Restlessness
- ⚡ Pain and heaviness in the chest and lungs
- ⚡ Tightness in the throat
- ⚡ Headaches
- ⚡ Stomach aches and disordered digestion
- ⚡ Changes in appetite and eating patterns
- ⚡ Difficulty falling asleep
- ⚡ Difficulty staying awake
- ⚡ Nightmares
- ⚡ Fatigue/ lack of energy/ lethargy
- ⚡ Increased sickness
- ⚡ Physical complaints
- ⚡ Slowed movements
- ⚡ Sensing the presence of the deceased
- ⚡ Visual, auditory or sense of touch of the deceased
- ⚡ Weight loss or gain
- ⚡ Taking care of others rather than self
- ⚡ Numbness and robotic behavior

Spiritual reactions

- ⚡ Changes in belief systems and values
- ⚡ Sense of hopelessness
- ⚡ Feeling abandoned by God or a spiritual community
- ⚡ Change in support system
- ⚡ Questioning faith and/or religious affiliation
- ⚡ Disconnect from self

- ⚡ Change in relationship with the Godhead or Divine Presence
- ⚡ Shift in prayer life
- ⚡ Shift in desire to worship and/or participate in ritual
- ⚡ Shift in priorities

The above are common, natural ways in which grief affects us.

The following thoughts and behaviors are cause for concern:

- ⚡ Depression
- ⚡ Eating disorders
- ⚡ Withdrawal
- ⚡ Destructive behavior
- ⚡ Recurring flashbacks
- ⚡ Substance abuse
- ⚡ Suicidal or homicidal thoughts
- ⚡ Risk taking behaviors

Please seek the counsel of a professional therapist or health care provider if your reaction to grief includes thoughts or behaviors that potentially put the health and welfare of yourself or others at risk.

To feel is to heal

Grief is a profoundly personal and internal experience, and it often has no external symptoms that are readily recognizable to others. We don't walk with a limp, for example, after our heart has been broken. As a yoga teacher, when I have offered special workshops for yoga and grief, I have often been surprised to have one of my regular students attend. More than once, I've had a student come to a yoga for grief workshop who had been attending my class on a weekly basis, yet I had no idea that her mother had died, or that she had lost a baby pre-term, or that someone in the family was critically or terminally ill. As convivial as the community is at the yoga studio, students choose how much or how little they reveal, and choose with whom they share their deepest sorrows.

Yoga is also deeply personal. A personal yoga practice tailored to you can "midwife" the deep, internal healing needed after an experience of loss. Choose the practices in this book that resonate with you. Try things out. Be curious. Notice what you feel. Be patient. Trust your intuition. Yoga practice helps us know, feel, and heal the emotional experiences recorded in every cell of our body. Healing requires that we honor our own edge and that we do not inflict pain on ourselves physically or psychologically. Yoga as a practice is aimed more toward self-acceptance, and less toward self-improvement. The practice begins with an acknowledgment of our own wholeness, our own innate goodness, and the intention to practice genuine compassion and love toward ourselves.

Attend to the basics of self-care

When we are grieving, or supporting a grieving person, we need to take care that our basic needs are being met. This is true at all times, but we need to be especially mindful when we are under any major life stress such as trauma or grief. Grief affects every system of the body, so eating nourishing food, drinking plenty of water, getting adequate sleep, creating space for conscious relaxation, and having time to play and do activities we enjoy are all aspects of a healing yoga practice. If you are a person of faith, prayer may be part of your yoga practice. We also need to connect with other people.

Resilience and self-care

Loss and life transition will test our resilience. Resilience isn't merely the ability to endure through difficult times and situations, but the ability to restore and renew our being through those situations and beyond. Good practices of self-care are important for restoration and renewal not only during grief and transition, but also for a lifetime of health and well-being. During periods of grief and transition, our habits of self-care may be compromised. These times in our life are an invitation to mindfully enter even more deeply into practices that nourish, heal and restore.

Grieving is an active process. It requires us to expend energy, and can feel like heavy work. The energy required for the active work of grieving may likely have to be withdrawn from some of the usual pursuits of life. You might consider letting some commitments go for a while, stepping back from some activities, and adjusting your work schedule to allow some breathing room and time and space for restoration, reflection, and solitude. Give yourself permission to create changes and treat yourself with the same love, compassion, understanding, and gentle care that you would extend toward a valued friend or loved one in a similar situation.

The following pages share suggestions that others have found useful in healthy, active grieving. Choose the ones that work for you, and feel free to invent your own methods.

"If I am not good to myself,
how can I expect anyone else to be good to me?"
~ **Maya Angelou**

SELF-CARE DO LIST

❀ **Learn to breathe again.** Allocate even five minutes every day to practice deep, diaphragmatic breathing. Deep breathing releases muscular tension, mental and emotional tension, and cleanses and restores the body. Changing a breathing habit or pattern rewires neuromuscular patterning. When we use the popular buzz phrases about the mind-body connection that is practiced in yoga, we're really talking about the breath-brain connection. The yogis say that when we change our breath, we change our mind, and when we change our mind, we change our life.

❀ **Go gently. Take the time that you need.** There is no deadline by which you should be "over" this. Grieving is not a process that helps us get over anything. Grieving is a process of integration and adaptation to a new way of being in the world.

❀ **Avoid making major decisions or taking on new responsibilities.**

❀ **Practice acceptance.** Grow to expect and accept some reduction in your usual efficiency, consistency, and productivity.

❀ **Speak your truth.** Talk regularly and truthfully about your grief and your memories with someone you trust to listen compassionately.

❀ **Tell the truth to yourself.** Check in with yourself. What am I experiencing right now, in this moment? What are my needs in this moment? Do I feel grounded, steady, healthy, and whole in this moment? Being honest with yourself is liberating. If you choose clarity and honesty, it will bring congruence to your thoughts, words, and actions, and help those around you feel at ease with the truth.

❀ **Be attentive to emotions.** Emotions are messengers, communicating information about our current state of wellness. Heavy emotions, sometimes called negative emotions, are the psyche's way of telling us that our needs are not being met. Anger may be a sign that we need to re-establish healthy limits and boundaries and keep our boundaries strong. Resentment can signal that we are not doing enough to care for ourselves. We don't always immediately know the message of our emotions, but we can practice paying attention to them.

❀ **Receive.** Accept help when it is offered.

❀ **Communicate clearly with those near you.** Ask for what you need. People are basically good, and the people around you can't read your mind. Many of them have no idea how to help or what to say. Don't take it personally. Ask them for what you need and teach them how to support a grieving person. Ask for it as directly as possible. This can be a great growing edge, especially for those of us who take pride in our personal independence. Tell friends and family what helps you and what does not. Most likely, they would like to help if they knew how.

- ❁ **Connect with others.** See a counselor, join a group, speak to a spiritual leader.

- ❁ **Connect with nature.** Walk in the woods, sit in the sun, plant a garden, play with a dog.

- ❁ **Eat. Exercise. Rest. Sleep.** Be especially attentive to maintaining healthy patterns of eating, sleeping, and exercise. Eat nourishing food. Exercise regularly and moderately. Maintain regular patterns of rest and sleep.

- ❁ **Practice conscious relaxation.** Do a restorative yoga pose and practice grounding and centering breath.

- ❁ **Read.** There are many helpful books on grief, and many useful resources on the Internet. Understanding grief may make it more manageable.

- ❁ **Plan.** Allow yourself to enjoy some good times without guilt. And allow yourself an exit strategy from a social gathering or freedom to cancel plans without guilt.

❀ **Avoid drugs and alcohol.** Mood altering chemicals can lengthen the grieving process by masking true emotions.

❀ **Remember.** Set aside specific time daily, weekly, seasonally, and annually for remembering and experiencing whatever feelings arise with the memories.

❀ **Plan for special days.** Feelings can be particularly intense on days such as holidays and anniversaries. Plan ahead to ensure your emotional and physical needs are met.

❀ **Pray.** Prayer is an ancient form of mind-body medicine. Create daily, weekly, and seasonal rhythms of personal prayer and prayer with a community if prayer brings you comfort, connection, and peace. Both believing that there is a Spirit to whom we can surrender our burdens and knowing that others are praying for us contribute positively to our healing process.

❀ **Make an altar or shrine for your memories or carry or wear a linking object.** Choose a keepsake that symbolically reminds you that you are in a period of grief, transition and personal growth. Or create a shrine in your home dedicated to your loved one and your grief process. There may come a time in the future when you no longer need this reminder. Then you can reverently let it go.

❀ **Take a yoga class.** There is healing power in community. Attend a class regularly and connect with other students.

✿ **Vent emotions in a healthy way.** That which we resist persists, and feelings that get buried alive will not die. Take a walk, or garden, or make music, join a choir, or do some vigorous yoga.

✿ **Choose entertainment carefully.** Certain TV shows, movies, and books can trigger and intensify already strong emotions.

✿ **Seek and find balance in every day.** Create time and space for yourself daily. Don't wait for the weekend or for your day off to take some "down time," away from screens and phones and electronics. Can't attend a yoga class? Do five minutes of yoga twice each day. Do a restorative pose, or a few sun salutations. Sit in quiet. Ask yourself, "What do I need today to nourish and heal myself? What do I need to feel balanced and whole?"

✿ **Give back.** Do something to help others. In addition to rituals of self-care, selfless service can be an effective way of overcoming sadness and lethargy and re-engaging in life. This may sound difficult and even counterintuitive, but caring for others when we are feeling deeply wounded is sometimes exactly what helps to lift us up and remind us of our connectedness with others.

✿ **Get a massage regularly.**

✿ **Take warm, leisurely baths**.

❀ **Keep a journal.** Write down your experiences, your feelings, and your life lessons. Healthy grieving can be a great teacher, and this period of your life may be a period of profound personal growth and transformation.

❀ **Forgive.** Forgive yourself. Your deceased loved one wouldn't want you to beat yourself up over something you said or did, or failed to say or do. Forgive the person or people who are gone from your life. Forgive the people around you who can't or won't acknowledge your grief and loss. If they are willing students, kindly and gently teach them how to support a grieving person. Everyone is going to die and everyone we love is someday going to die, so knowing how to grieve and how to support those who mourn is an important part of being human.

There is no substitute for a supportive community

The experience of grief or bereavement can make us feel isolated. We might think we're the only person on the planet experiencing deep sadness and going through great difficulty. Having a circle of support, companions on the journey, eases the pain of grief and helps us heal. Do not underestimate the healing power of community. During this fragile period of life, we need a safe space and permission to be as we are. We need compassion. We need caring companions. We need to be seen, heard, and touched. We need humor and laughter. In addition to developing a personal yoga practice, finding or creating a healing community with persons who share the experience of grief and who will share the practice of yoga will enhance and sweeten the healing process. We all need someone to hold the light for us when the darkness seems frightening. Knowing that we are connected, not alone, gives us hope. We also need to give hope and love and encouragement to others. This helps to open and heal our hearts.

Serenity, now!

The Serenity Prayer by the American theologian Reinhold Niebuhr (1892–1971) is the credo of many 12-step programs. This prayer is also very appropriate in *Honoring Loss*. The best known form of the prayer is:

Grant me the serenity to accept the
things I cannot change,
The courage to change the things I can,
And the wisdom to know the difference.

In the experience of grief, healing ultimately comes through acceptance and surrender, which is also described as grace. And, paradoxically, surrender is a choice, an act of will, and requires tremendous courage. Serenity is a practice. We don't have to do it perfectly at all times.

In a memorably hilarious *Seinfeld* episode, Frank Costanza learns the phrase "Serenity, now!" from a self-help recording and shouts it desperately in moments of tribulation. Shouting out a *mantra* may be one way to fortify our will and help us grow in grace. Yoga tradition offers many wise suggestions for practices to strengthen our resolve and our ability to let go of things that are beyond our control. The *yamas* and *niyamas*, the first two limbs of classical yoga, are a good foundation for practicing will and grace.

"As the wind loves to call things to dance,
May your gravity be lightened by grace."
~ John O'Donohue

The System of Yoga

Classical yoga, or eight-limbed yoga

The sage Patanjali is considered to be the father of classical yoga. The age-old text, the *Yoga Sutras*, a set of teachings which describes the practice of *Rāja Yoga* as a tree with eight limbs, is attributed to Patanjali. The eight limbs of classical yoga represent eight steps on the path toward the light of wisdom. The first two limbs are *yama* and *niyama*, usually translated from the Sanskrit as restraint and non-restraint. The *yamas* guide the yogi's attitude toward living in right relationship with the self and others; the *niyamas* are a set of self-observances, or qualities to cultivate for purification and upright living. The spirit of the *yamas* and *niyamas* is found in all world religions. In the *Yoga Sutras* we see how the philosophy of yoga extends beyond the limits of any one religious sect or belief system.

BE GENTLE WITH YOURSELF and other practices of will and grace

Practices for living through grief, transition, and loss: Yamas and niyamas for the grieving

I like to think of the *yamas* and *niyamas* as practices of will and grace. They are not commandments, nor are they a list of "shoulds" and "should nots." Please don't should on yourself. The *yamas* and *niyamas* are practices to cultivate in the interest of a life that is more balanced, whole, and free. They address the totality of life, and they begin with an attitude of non-violence, gentleness, and compassion toward ourselves and all beings. Following is one possible interpretation of the *yamas* and *niyamas* which may resonate in the hearts and minds of those who grieve. The Sanskrit and English translation of each *yama* or *niyama* is included here. After, you will find a set of questions which you might use as a journaling practice or, if you are working with this text with a friend or a group, you might consider them as discussion questions.

Yamas: Relational practices with others

Living in right relationship with and others and the external world.

By practicing the five *yamas*, we may grow in self-awareness, peace, and equanimity. Here is a brief description of each *yama*, with some suggestions about how to begin practicing them as part of your healing journey, or noticing that you are already practicing them today.

1

Ahimsa ~ Non-violence

A state of mind and way of being that is without enmity or aggression. Practice kindness, compassion, empathy, and non-harming.

In Sanskrit the prefix a- means "not," and *himsa* means "harming, doing violence, injuring or killing." The practice of doing no harm to anyone is universally recognized as essential in all the healing arts, and true non-violence is foundational to yoga practice. Begin with genuine non-violence towards yourself. Be kind and gentle with yourself. Treat yourself at least as kindly as you would treat a beloved friend who is working through a difficult time and situation. Allow yourself to feel, without passing judgment on your feelings. Practice self-compassion, serenity, and self-acceptance. Move away from thoughts or language that is self-critical or criticizes others. "Should haves," "could haves," or "would haves" are not only useless, these thoughts often create harm. Let them go.

Perfectionism and non-violence

Be wary of the perfectionism demon. Perfectionism is a subtle and dangerous form of self-hatred. Yoga as a path is first concerned with self-acceptance before self-improvement. To move through the process of grief we must start where we are, acknowledging the truth and reality of the present. Right where you are right now is the perfect place to begin this process. Be gentle with yourself. Be gentle with others and all sentient beings and the universe. Practice self-care. Accept your own limits and the limitations of others.

Choose kindness as a *sadhana*

Choosing kindness can sound so warm and fuzzy, but as a real life practice it is very challenging, especially when we are physically or emotionally suffering or hurting. Choosing kindness, both for ourselves and others, isn't just being "nice," and the practice of *ahimsa* does not ask us to be a human doormat for the violence and harmful deeds of others.

Choose kindness, non-violence, and non-aggression as a practice. The Sanskrit word for practice is *sadhana*, which can also be translated as sacrifice. Choosing kindness is indeed a sacrifice; it does means that we have to let go of any urge to retaliate or seek revenge when we are wronged or mistreated. Yet choosing kindness doesn't require us to be silent or unresponsive when we are being harmed or when others around us are being mistreated or abused. In fact, our silence and apathy in the face of injustice and violence may make us complicit in the harmful conduct of others. Albert Einstein once said, "The world is a dangerous place, not because of those who do evil, but because of those who look on and do nothing."

As we choose kindness as a *sadhana* we become advocates for the common good and well-being of all. Sometimes we must sacrifice our concerns about our own reputation, and speak up against the violence around us. What will others think of us or say about us if we take a stand? The practice of yoga is concerned about our personal character, not our reputation. What others say about us is their business; they will have to live with the consequence of their gossip or malevolent words. What we think and say and do is our business. We are developing and living into our own, authentic character.

Beginner's Mind

We come to the practice of *ahimsa*, and our whole yoga practice, for that matter, with the mind of a beginner, for as the Zen saying attributed to Shunryu Suzuki goes, "In the beginner's mind there are many possibilities. In the expert's mind there are few." The idea of having the mindset of a beginner refers to having an attitude of discovery, exploration, eagerness, openness, and lack of preconceptions or biases when studying a subject or practicing a discipline, even when studying at an advanced level. We approach the study and practice as though it is brand new every day. In this respect, having a beginner's mind is actually very advanced.

Begin the practice of *ahimsa* by mindfully observing your own thoughts and words, spoken and unspoken, every day. Keep watch over your mind and mouth. Consciously choose thoughts, words, and actions that demonstrate acceptance, understanding, and real love for yourself and others.

Using a process similar to the *Examen* found in the spiritual exercises of St. Ignatius Loyola, you might take inventory at the end of each day:

- *In thoughtful reflection, note the events of the day for which you are particularly grateful. You may choose to write your thoughts in a journal.*
- *Examine the events of the day which were particularly challenging or could have gone better.*
- *Forgive yourself and others for any harm or wrongdoing that occurred that day.*
- *Resolve to begin the practice again tomorrow. Ask for the grace to practice well.*

Practice non-violent communication. Practice loving kindness. Practice forgiveness. When you have been wronged, try shifting the focus from blaming the perpetrator, and instead practice self-understanding and self-compassion. Let go of resentment and rage for the sake of your own health and well-being. Set yourself free from those heavy burdens. Honor yourself and your experience, and be gentle with yourself.

Questions about *ahimsa*

- 🏵 *Give examples of violence toward the self.*

- 🏵 *Can you create space for all of your emotions, even feelings that are uncomfortable or unfamiliar? If you are aware of feelings of anger, hatred, or jealousy, what can you do with those feelings for the benefit of yourself and others? Can you practice non-violence and compassion toward yourself and others?*

- 🏵 *Why is the practice of non-violent communication so important?*

- 🏵 *Can you reach out to someone else and ask for support in practicing* ahimsa *today?*

- 🏵 *How carefully do you choose your car, your cell phone, your clothing, your shoes, and your food? The practice of* ahimsa *invites us to be at least that choosy regarding the thoughts we think, the words we say, and the actions we perform. Can you be very particular about the thoughts you choose today?*

- 🏵 *What is something you can do today or each day to practice compassion toward yourself?*

2

Satya ~ Non-lying

**Practice truthfulness. When you speak, speak
about things that are true. Let your speech
elevate the universe.**

The word *sat*, in Sanskrit, means "true; that which exists; that which is." *Satya* is usually translated as "truthfulness." What is truth? So many messages are available to us about the world and its peoples, about human experiences and feelings. Are they all true? As you move through the process of grief, allow yourself to be truthful. Embrace your own truth, and speak it kindly when it feels right to do so.

Take nothing personally. People often say awkward, clumsy things in their efforts to console or advise the grieving, so cut other people a little slack. Let's face it: people don't always know what they're saying.

Cut yourself some slack, too. Grieving is hard, exhausting work. You don't have to do it perfectly. Notice your feelings and emotions. There is truth in what you feel. You are not your feelings; you are greater than any one feeling or experience. Yet feelings carry wisdom. Notice the physical sensations in your belly, your heart, your throat, your body. Tension and discomfort in the body is normal during periods of high stress and personal suffering. You don't need to pretend that you feel any differently than you do, or that your current situation is not difficult. No one benefits from you pretending that you're "fine." You don't owe anyone a fake smile. And maybe it's true that, in many ways, you are "fine." Is life ever 100% good or bad? Allow yourself time and space to take a truthful inventory of the good as well as the not-so-good. If it's the truth, it's okay to think or say, "I'm not liking this very much right now." The practice of *satya* is subordinate to the practice of *ahimsa*, so if words are harmful, even if they're true, they are best left unsaid.

The power of words

I recently received an anonymous hate letter, my first in the more than 40 years that I've worked for the public in human service professions. For the most part, my work has been a rich and joyous experience, and I have felt truly privileged to do it. It has also required personal growth and learning. I haven't done everything perfectly. There were occasions when I was more reactive than responsive to the needs of the people I serve. There were times when difficult conversations didn't go well, when my words and actions were poorly chosen or misunderstood. I'd say that's called "being human." Truthfully, some of my worst life moments have been in times of great duress and grief. Is grief an excuse? No. But I can forgive myself and acknowledge that I am a work in progress and capable of doing better.

The anonymous author of the hate letter didn't refer to any specific incident. She resorted to character assassination.

(I say "she" because the writer referred to herself as a mother.) She said she'd known me for 15 years, and claimed that I was not valued by anyone and hated by many people. Her toxic language made me feel sick. It's called "the poison pen" for a reason.

As I reflected on the experience, I actually felt sorry for the sender. What kind of a person types a letter, prints a letter, puts it in an envelope, prints a typed address label, puts the address label and a stamp on the envelope, and mails the letter? That's no small effort for the sake of harming someone.

Is it possible that, in the past, in subtle and insidious ways, I have actually assassinated my own character and sabotaged myself with negative self-talk, harmful thoughts and demeaning judgments about my own inadequacy or personal value? Have I beaten myself up for my own mistakes, not allowing myself to be human, and denying my ability to grow beyond a low moment?

Hate speech and gossip is damaging. In some religious traditions, gossip is considered to be among the most deadly sins. Words matter. Words, both those spoken silently to ourselves and out loud to others, matter. Once those words have been thought or spoken, they cannot be retrieved. Once a rumor, a "secret story," or a bit of gossip leaves our lips, we cannot know where it ends up, and we can never get it back.

Non-violent communication encourages us to own and examine our thoughts and feelings, and consciously choose words that are truthful, useful, and that build up people and relationships, not tear them down with insults and degradation.

Moderation of thought, truthfulness in word, and kindness in action are practices. Like learning to play a musical instrument, it takes time and dedication to develop consistency and skill in this practice. The practice of non-violent communication is a topic worthy of exploration in its own right, and a few very fine manuals have been written on this subject.

Be gentle with yourself and others in the thoughts you think and the words you say. If the truth is pleasant, speak it. If the truth is unpleasant, speak it kindly, without creating harm or damage. Do your best to grieve truthfully, and in a manner that doesn't harm yourself or others. This will leave no further scars on your already wounded heart. Advocate for your own needs and stand in your truth.

Pay attention to the stories you are telling yourself about your current situation. You are more than your story or your current circumstances.

Keep in mind: a story may or may not be true.

Truth-check practice

Periodically check in with yourself. How do you feel? Let the honest answer arise from within you. Learn to recognize the emotions that may lead you to twist the truth. Learn to recognize your personal "triggers." Notice if feelings of loneliness, waves of sadness, even sensations of hunger and fatigue, make you more vulnerable or prone to reactivity. Can you give yourself space and a little time out when you need it?

Check in with yourself at the end of a day. When did you practice kindness and truth today? Lay down the day each time the sun sets. Let the past be the past and forgive anyone who has misspoken to you. Forgive others, not necessarily because they deserve it, but because you do. The burden of anger and resentment is heavy. Anger can be a signal that you need to establish stronger boundaries. Resentment can be a reminder to invest more energy into doing good things for yourself, nourishing and restoring your being.

Practice silence

The practice of keeping silent can be a useful practice for cultivating truthfulness. Spend a few minutes each day in silence. Find a comfortable position reclined, seated, standing or walking. Eliminate distractions, and just breathe. If the mind begins to "talk," invite the thoughts to pause, and bring awareness to the simplicity of your breath.

Love letter

Write a letter to yourself. Acknowledge your current suffering and pain, and enumerate all the admirable qualities that you are demonstrating as you do the very difficult work of grieving.

A story of letting go and *satya* practice from my life

I colored my hair for about two decades of my life. It began as an artistic, aesthetic exercise. In my 30s, I realized I could "augment" the tone of certain hues in my hair and create almost any look I wanted. I also discovered a couple of looks I didn't want. Overall, I didn't have a bad batting average. But as I approached my 50s, I started noticing the clash between the softness of my salt and pepper roots and the strong color of the cosmetically manipulated strands. I was struggling to find a hair color that complemented my skin tone, warming without overwhelming.

The month before my 49th birthday, I thought I had found a great look – light brown hair with summery highlights. Then I received in the mail some professional photographs of our beautiful family. We were all dressed in shades of blue and grey, posed against a similarly subtle background. My husband looked so distinguished. White and silver streaked his curly hair. My young adult son looked athletic and smart, his brown hair trimmed within a quarter inch of his scalp, the strong features of his handsome face shining.

Then there was this woman. Wait. Was her hair orange? Who, at least on this planet, has orange hair? The contrast was startling. The hair went with absolutely nothing else in the photo – not the background, not the clothing, not the woman's face and eyes.

I walked to the bathroom and looked in the mirror. A strand of white was growing in around my face. For the first time since the "saltiness" of my hair had started to reveal itself, I thought to myself, "That's not unattractive." Really? This was news.

I'd been racing against these stealthily encroaching greys for years, thinking I could outwit if not outrun them. Now, I noticed a shift in my perspective and I wondered if my grey hair and I could become friends.

The truth be told, I was weary of the time and money spent in the salon searching for that "perfect" look. Years ago a trip to the salon was like a vacation, precious pampered "me time." Now I'd rather have a massage or a real vacation. I was also never fond of the stains on the skin around my hairline that sometimes lasted for days after the whole color exercise was complete. The dyed hair no longer looked aesthetic or artsy as it might have in my younger days. It just looked dyed. In that moment, I decided I was done. I was ready to let it go.

I argued with myself. Then I thought, "What's the worst that could happen? I won't like my natural color and I'll go back to coloring it. Meanwhile, I'm going to go for it." I didn't have to push it away to let it go; I could begin by simply letting it be. I started to announce my decision to my family, friends, and coworkers. The more I said it out loud, the more it strengthened my resolve. Even my hairdresser affirmed my decision. "It'll look beautiful. I think you'll be very happy with the results." She was an ally and coach who supported me the whole way.

The transition to my natural hair color, which took more than a full year, required patience and perseverance. By no means was it the most difficult thing I'd ever done. It is, after all, just hair. But it was and is MY hair.

Navigating serious grief, transition, and loss has helped me to grow to become a strong person who knows and speaks her truth. Allowing my hair to return to its natural color was a personal choice that I made to practice *satya*. And I've been very happy with that choice.

Questions about *Satya*

- 🏵 *Describe examples of speech that elevates the universe. How can our speech lift up the overall condition of life, making the world a better place? Give examples of speech that denigrates the universe.*

- 🏵 *Notice how you feel after conversations. What is the emotional and energetic "residue" of the conversation?*

- 🏵 *Describe a situation when you found it difficult to be truthful. Why was it hard? When you chose to speak your truth or conceal your truth, what were the results?*

❀ *How do you feel about gossip? How does it make you feel when you gossip about another person, or when you hear that someone has gossiped about you? When you hear others gossiping, how can you respond in a clear, calm, and effective way?*

❀ *The teachings of some religious traditions seem to suggest that pride is evil, but pride is not inherently damaging; arrogance and hubris are harmful. Of what life accomplishments are you honestly and truthfully proud? What achievements in your life have helped you express the truth of your Being? How are you actively working in your life to embrace the truth of your own innate goodness?*

❀ *People are sometimes attached to their personal truths around the mystery of death and loss. What are the results of this attachment? When others say awkward or even hurtful things, can you practice compassion towards them and towards yourself and forgive?*

❀ *Describe an aspect of the grief experience about which you find it very difficult to be truthful.*

3

Asteya ~ Non-coveting and non-stealing

Practice abundance.

The Sanskrit word *steya* means "stealing," and again the prefix *a-* means "not." The practice of non-stealing and non-coveting includes not stealing or coveting other people's ideas, words, property, or happiness. When our hearts are aching and broken, it can be very difficult to avoid the temptation of longing for someone else's life. We don't really wish them harm or want to rob them of their happiness; we just might wonder, "Why did this sorrow or tragedy occur in my life? Why does that individual appear to have the perfect life?"

Things are not always as they appear. Avoid comparing your insides to other people's outsides. You might even notice that, if you make such comparisons, you "steal" from yourself your own potential contentment. Practice acceptance of your questions and feelings. Practice gentleness with your own longings and desires. Don't completely deny your desires; rather, notice them. Your longings and wishes may lead you to a greater understanding of your personal calling and deeper connection with your true Self.

Practice gratitude as a habit of the mind and heart. This, too, can be very difficult when life seems bleak. Practice living in the present moment, for in the present moment, all needs are met. Affirm small pleasures – the good taste of a cup of tea, the crisp colors in nature, the leisure of a walk in the sunshine, the beautiful sounds in a favorite piece of music. Complete the "pleasure loop" between the mind and the body by saying out loud to yourself things like, "Mmm, this food tastes good" or "this warm coat feels cozy." Saying it out loud will reinforce in your own mind the idea that life is good.

If you find it useful, keep a gratitude journal. At the end of each day, make a list of events or moments for which you are grateful. Try to come up with at least one unique thing for which you are grateful every day. You may find that this practice helps you be on the look out for new blessings each day.

Some of my students have mentioned to me that they keep gratitude jars. Every day, they write down on small strips of paper events or things for which they are grateful that day. They place the strips in the jar. When they're feeling down, they pull a strip out of the jar to remember one of the many, random blessings of life.

Above all, cultivate a spirit of gratitude for your unique, precious human life. Within you, there is a life force, unique in all the world, that you are bringing to birth in the process of your grief and your life. When we covet someone else's life, we steal from ourselves the opportunity to discover our own unique purpose.

Practice giving. Participate in the healing power of community by giving of your time, your treasure and your talent as you are able. As you connect in a positive way to other people through the material world, sharing your personal resources, you cultivate joy for yourself and others.

Questions about *Asteya*

- ✺ *Why would claiming someone else's truth, words or ideas to be our own without living it, experiencing it and internalizing it, be harmful? Who might it harm?*

- ✺ *Give examples of stealing, other than blatant robbery, that go on in the world every day? How does this stealing affect us all?*

- ✺ *What practices might you cultivate to balance asteya, and create a sense of inner wealth, even as you move through this grieving process?*

"Don't compare your insides to
someone else's outsides."
~ **Moya McGinn Mathews**

Gratitude "stretch" for balancing *asteya* and celebrating abundance

This "stretch" isn't a yoga pose; it's a journal exercise, and practicing it can lift your spirits, no matter where you begin. If you're feeling low, it may lift the heaviness from your heart. If you're feeling great, it might lift you up even more.

In your journal, or on a blank sheet of paper, write the numbers one through 50 from top to bottom on the left hand side of the page. Then list 50 things that you like, love, or appreciate about your life. Write the numbers first, so you don't quit after the first few easy and obvious responses that come to mind. For example, in my life, I am grateful for my family, my education, good health, a close circle of friends, a yoga teaching job that I love, and a comfortable and cozy home. My "top five" come to mind without any real effort on my part. When I stretch a bit, I remember that I am grateful to drink fresh, hot coffee every morning. I am grateful for modern plumbing and a hot shower. I am grateful to be able to walk outside and breath fresh, clean air. I'm fortunate to live in a city with many opportunities and very little pollution. My list could go on. What's on your list?

4

Brahmacharya ~ Non-excess

Practice respect and reverence.

Brahmacharya literally means "behavior which leads to the Creator." Because we are created in the image of the Creator, the practice of *brahmacharya* is the practice of living our lives in a manner that is in harmony with our true Self, with our own innate goodness. In some Indian religions it refers to a monastic lifestyle characterized by sexual continence or complete abstinence. We are not all monks, so a broader understanding of *brahmacharya* encourages us to travel our life's journey with a godly purpose and godly consciousness, to assert self-control and mastery over our own creative force, to practice reverence and respect for our own body, our own life, and to harmonize our own creative life force with the larger whole.

When we cultivate an attitude of deep self-respect and demonstrate reverence for life and our creative power, we are practicing *brahmacharya*. This includes protecting our energy and conserving it for higher purposes, such as a spiritual purpose or the purpose of our own personal transformation. It also involves avoiding mindless chatter or activities with no clear purpose.

When we are grieving, we have the opportunity to re-assess how we want to spend our time and energy and with whom we want to spend it. The practice of *brahmacharya* allows us to consciously choose relationships and creative activities that are purposeful, fulfilling and emotionally satisfying. As we differentiate creativity from mere busyness or outright chaos, we may come to a renewed sense of wonder in ourselves and a clearer sense of our life's purpose.

Relationships often shift during periods of grief; as we change and transform through the process of grief, we will find that some relationships fall away from our lives and new relationships develop. Our profession or vocation may also change as we re-define our priorities and make new choices regarding how we will use our life's creative power. As we become more precise in our decisions regarding our use of our personal power, we begin to live a powerful, dynamic life.

The cultivation of mastery over one's own personal power includes the practice of rest and relaxation. No one can live a purposeful and dynamic life without incorporating meaningful ways to rest – to renew and restore the soul. Healing requires rest. Be gentle with yourself.

Questions about _Brahmacharya_

- 🏵 _Grieving requires tremendous energy. Whether we are holding and restraining emotion or releasing emotion, the emotional energy of grief can be heavy, and carrying it can be exhausting. Where do you find regular sabbath, or rest, in your life? What daily, weekly and seasonal rituals do you or can you incorporate into your life to renew and restore your soul?_

- 🏵 _What books and magazines have you read lately? What movies have you watched? How do you feel after reading them or watching them?_

- 🏵 _You might choose a verse of scripture or poetry or a quote that you find meaningful and recite it as part of your morning routine to help direct the energy of your daily life. Later in this book, we will further address the concept of_ san kalpa, _or sacred intention, and you might formulate a statement of personal intention that becomes part of your daily yoga practice._

5

Aparigraha ~ Non-grasping, non-greed, non-attachment, non-possessiveness

Practice letting it be.

Graha means "to grasp" and *pari* means "things": *aparigraha* means "not grasping things." The spirit of *aparigraha* suggests that the whole world and all that is in it is available for our enjoyment and for our use as needed, but not necessarily for our ownership. *Aparigraha* is similar to the biblical value of stewardship. We make good use of the things that come to us without becoming attached to them.

I personally like nice things. My happiness is not dependent on owning nice things, though I do enjoy the nice things that I have available to me. I also recognize that I am in a very privileged position, because I know with some certainty that all my basic needs will be met every day. I used to enjoy shopping, not only for essentials, but for all sorts of things. After my husband, Chad, died, shopping became a nearly therapeutic pastime for me. I enjoyed putting on nice clothes, washing my face, grooming my hair, going out in public, looking at pretty things, and socializing with the people who worked in the stores that I visited. Sometimes I bought things that I didn't need, though I never created financial harm for myself or my family. One of the aspects of shopping that I most appreciated was that, as a customer in a store, I could maintain a certain amount of anonymity, revealing or concealing as much or as little of my personal story as I chose. In so many arenas of my life – at my office, my church, my son's school – I was known as a widow, or as Chad's widow. As a shopper, I could drop that story and identity and just be another 30-something woman at the mall.

Stories and identities are tricky. We can get attached not only to things, but also to the people and the way of life we love, creating an identity for ourselves around a certain way of life that is very comfortable and familiar. It happens. We become accustomed to a certain pattern of living that includes our loved ones and certain activities and schedules. We find a sense of security in that way of life. A new, unfamiliar way of life may force us to redefine our identity, and that can be very uncomfortable.

Aparigraha and transition and loss

I remember my son's senior year of high school being a particularly difficult time for me. He was healthy and well and thriving, yet as I anticipated the life transition that would include his graduation and leaving home to go away to college, I felt deeply sad. That year, we celebrated many milestone events, and I remember feeling sad with the thought, "This is the last time we'll do this together."

It is certainly true that life would never be the same. But what did I want for my son? I wanted him to have the confidence to venture into the world as a happy, independent, and capable adult. My hopes as a mother were being fulfilled. Together, we had been preparing for this transition for 18 years, and still, I found it difficult. As he grew and matured and made courageous decisions, my identity and my way of life were shifting. Once he left for college, it took time and courage for me to adjust to a new stage of life as an empty nester. Now, years later, we have all found happiness, and are living beautiful lives filled with a sense of purpose. My life as his mother was changed, not ended. His life as a young man is being fulfilled.

Healing requires time and sacrifice. Grasping for the past or clinging to former plans can create obstacles in our efforts to move through grief and life transition toward acceptance. If we want to live a life that is healthy and whole, and the way we're currently thinking and living does not allow space for our wholeness, then we need to change our thoughts and our life. As author Joseph Campbell said, "We must let go of the life we have planned, so as to accept the one that is waiting for us."

What is waiting for us is mysterious and unknown, and real emotional security is found in our ability to live with the knowledge that everything is impermanent and we are in control of very little. The yogis seem to tell us, "Be unattached; don't hold on, don't cling; just let it go." Sometimes letting it go is too much to ask. Letting it go might feel like effort, or as though we're trying to push the experience or the feeling away. Try letting it be.

Again, remember the famous Serenity Prayer: "Grant me the serenity to accept the things I cannot change, courage to change the things I can, and wisdom to know the difference." One moment at a time, one breath at a time, can we find the ability to be at ease with the vulnerability of "letting it be?"

Aparigraha and non-competition

Practice non-competition, even in the arena of grief. Avoid comparing yourself to others, comparing your life to others' lives, or comparing your grief to others' grief. No one's grief is more than, less than, or equal to your own. Your story is unique. And everyone else's story is unique. Again, beware of comparing your insides to someone else's outsides. We cannot know from our external observations of another person what that individual is experiencing internally.

Rebuilding after loss

When we lose something or someone and our identification with that person or thing or relationship must change, we have the opportunity to rebuild ourselves. When we are able to transform grief, we can reshape our perception of reality so that it more authentically resonates with our true nature. To do so, we must nourish ourselves. How are you nourishing yourself through this grieving process?

Practice: breath and mindfulness as pain management

Spend a few minutes daily just being aware of your own being. Use your breath as a tool, an anchor for your attention to keep you grounded in the present moment. You don't have to control it. Just feel its sensations. Be present to the flow of the breath, in and out. The body is a container for the breath. Notice how the shape of the body changes with each inhalation and exhalation. Breathe into any pain or tension to dissolve it and move through it. As the breath leaves the body, it returns freely. Our breath is precious; without it we die. The practice of letting the breath go and letting the breath be is a practice of trust and surrender.

"You can't push a wave onto the shore
any faster than the ocean brings it in."
~ Susan Strasberg

Questions about *Aparigraha*

🪷 *What do you consider a need? Do you have access to all your needs?*

🪷 *Have some of your needs become compromised during this period of grief? Have you noticed yourself compensating for those needs by over-indulging in other ways? This question is not to create guilt or self-punishment in the form of self-judgment; it's only to bring awareness to a behavior pattern, if it exists. Awareness of patterns or habits that do not serve our health, well-being, and happiness is the first step in halting the behavior and moving toward replacing it with a behavior that is truly life-giving.*

🪷 *Are there activities that you previously enjoyed and now miss due to the loss of a loved one? Without rushing the grief process, is there something new waiting for you that you might receive into your life for your enjoyment and nourishment?*

🪷 *Do you enjoy shopping? Shopping can be a pleasant reason to dress up and go out of the house. It's also not uncommon to buy things we don't need when we're grieving, as an attempt to fill the void. What items have you purchased in the past few months? Make a list. How do you feel about those purchases now?*

Niyamas ~ Relational practices with myself

Tuning in to the light within.

The five niyamas are tools for personal growth. Practicing them every day may help to cultivate happiness and self-confidence.

1

Saucha ~ Cleanliness

Practice cleanliness or purity.

Saucha means "purification or cleanliness." The practice of yoga includes many techniques for cleansing, renewing, and purifying the physical body, and also for cleansing and purifying the mind, the emotions, our material environment, and the chronological space that we create for our living.

Our physical body

The cleanliness and purity that yogis promote is not mere external cleanliness, although practices of purity certainly include washing and bathing. Washing and bathing can be emotionally and energetically useful, too. Have you ever noticed that after a significant emotional release, washing your face, or even putting a clean, moist, cool or warm cloth on your face helps to move the energy out and through you and allows the past experience to rest behind you?

After a particularly hard day or vigorous physical work, have you observed that a shower or bath eases tension and cleanses not only your body but shifts your energy and mood as well? When you take a shower or bath, take a moment to be aware of the effects. Enjoy the sensations of clear, clean water on your skin and hair. You might use fragrances or essential oils that help you feel grounded or invigorated, and scents that soothe your nervous system. Bathing can also be a gratitude practice. Marvel at the wonder of modern plumbing, if you're fortunate enough to have it: hot water comes directly out of a wall!

The grieving yogi seeks both physical and internal cleanliness to support emotional clarity, health, and wholeness. When we are grieving or in a post-traumatic state, our adrenals may be working overtime and our immune system may be taxed. Now, more than ever, we need to honor our body as a sacred temple for our emotions and our life experience. Take a personal inventory of your diet, your sleep habits, and your physical environment. Are you eating sufficient amounts of clean, whole food and consuming sugar, alcohol, or caffeine only minimally if at all?

Our physical space
Does your home environment support healthy practices of rest and restoration? Is clutter or the remaining possessions of a loved one who is no longer in your life because of death or the termination of a relationship creating stress for you

in your home, even making it difficult to rest and sleep well? If so, can you find a trustworthy friend or two to help you clean the space in a respectful way? Renewing our physical environment after the death of a loved one or the end of a relationship can be very difficult and also very renewing. It is a way to acknowledge the reality of the loss and create space for something new. Create a clean and a comfortable space for yourself where you can relax and feel at home and at peace.

Our chronological space

How clean is your calendar? Do you have time and space in your life to emotionally digest the events of your day? If your work or social life requires you to commute between activities and appointments, do you have sufficient time to travel safely and unhurriedly? Make periodic "check ins" with yourself throughout the day. Wiggle your toes. Notice your breath. Tune in to sensations and emotions.

Emotional and energetic cleanliness

Notice how you feel after watching certain movies or television shows. If they leave you feeling agitated, tense, or upset, considered removing those environmental and emotional "toxins" from your life. Notice your thoughts and your environment. Are there things in your thoughts or environment that you can eliminate to create more cleanliness and clarity? Is there anything you can add – a positive thought, a flower, a photograph – to make your mental and physical environment more pleasant or soothing?

The most powerful practice for the purpose of purification is the practice of rest. When we sleep or practice conscious relaxation, the body cleanses and restores itself. Do you have an uncluttered physical space in your home that supports the practice of relaxation and rest? Is your bedroom a space that helps you be at ease and supports your practice of rest?

Nature bathing

If at all possible, spend time outdoors in nature and bathe your senses in its beauty. The Navajo Indians have a practice called walking in beauty. This prayer, "In Beauty I Walk," is from the Navajo Way Blessing Ceremony:

> With beauty before me I walk,
> With beauty behind me I walk,
> With beauty above me I walk,
> With beauty around me I walk.

I would add, "With beauty inside me I walk." Even those parts of me that don't feel beautiful right now are essential for my becoming my best self and fulfilling my highest purpose. I am beautiful.

Questions about *Saucha*

❀ *Think of an example of a clear decision that you've made, choosing what you wanted and eliminating what you did not want. What was the result?*

❀ *Does your current schedule, diet, and home and work environment support you in living a healthy, balanced life?*

❀ *Are there things that you can do to eliminate clutter from your life, including the clutter of unnecessary activities? You might go through your weekly calendar and eliminate two or three things per week that you don't really have to do. You might clean a closet or a drawer and give away material possessions you're no longer using and no longer need.*

2

Santosha ~ Contentment

Practice contentment.

The word *santosha* means "contentment," or could also be translated as "delight, happiness, or joy." The idea of practicing contentment or practicing happiness is alien in a culture dedicated to trying to make us believe that happiness comes from things outside of us.

The message of the cultural media and advertising machine is, "When I get the perfect car/ partner/ house/ haircut/ or have the perfect physique/ job/ income/ children, then I will be happy. I am not enough." The message of yoga is that contentment is our nature. Happiness is our natural state of balance; it is already within of us. We are enough. The message of the psalmist resonates here: "You formed my inmost being; you knit me in my mother's womb. I praise you, because I am wonderfully made; wonderful are your works! My very self you know." (Psalms 139:13-14)

When we're grieving, happiness can seem pretty unattainable. After my husband died, I remember telling a couple of my best friends that, "I don't think I'm going to be very much fun to be around for a long time." Being true friends, they told me that it was not my job to entertain them or make their life fun. They gave me permission to show up as I was, not as I thought I was supposed to be.

Santosha does not deny or judge emotions. Too often we judge emotions – our own or others' – because we don't know what else to do with them. Emotions are important; they are messengers of our needs. We all have needs. That doesn't make us "needy," it makes us human. We don't always hear or understand what our emotions are trying to communicate to us. The practice of listening for the message requires trust – trust in ourselves and in a Greater Power or Spirit.

Santosha also does not deny the reality of suffering. All humans, all sentient beings, suffer. To dismiss the reality of this suffering with pithy advice to "be happy" or "be grateful" would be cruel. In the face of real suffering, we practice real compassion toward ourselves and others. *Santosha* acknowledges that there is a deep, abiding contentment present within us, even in the face of suffering. It's a mystery; feelings of contentment and feelings of discomfort and suffering can exist within us, side by side.

Santosha is a practice, and like any practice, the practice of yoga or the practice of santosha doesn't require perfection. That's why we call it a practice. Practice requires us to make mistakes. Sometimes we even make a mess. So we practice forgiveness and compassion. We are all a work in progress, and sometimes when the work feels the hardest, we're making the most significant progress.

Being authentic in the messiness of our life and emotions is part of being balanced and whole. Learning to be at home and content in the murkiness of life is a yogic practice. Cry or laugh when you can. Have fun, laugh, and laugh at yourself kindly. Find time and space to safely release the emotions that are part of the life experience we call "grief."

Practice self-care. Notice activities that allow you to feel happy and lose yourself in the activity – making or listening to music, dancing freestyle in the kitchen, singing in a choir, gardening, biking, yoga. Flow activities help us connect with contentment, which is our true nature. Find a life-enriching activity that you love to do and do it often – daily, if possible.

Questions about *Santosha*

> 🏵 *How are the practice of* santosha *(contentment) and the practice of* ahimsa *(non-violence) connected?*

> 🏵 *Give an example of a time when you practiced real compassion toward yourself. What was the result?*

> 🏵 *Describe an activity that helps you cultivate contentment and joy. Describe a recent moment when you experienced contentment.*

Final three niyamas

The final three *niyamas* constitute the threefold path of *Kriya Yoga*, the yoga of transformation and spiritual evolution. We could consider these *niyamas* as the Great Serenity Prayer of Yoga. *Isvara pranidhana* (surrender) is the serenity to accept to the things we cannot change, *tapas* (fiery determination) is the courage to change the things we can, and *svadhyaya* (self-study) is the wisdom to know the difference.

3

Tapas ~ Fire, heat, self-discipline

Do your practice. Do your work.

The literal translation of the Sanskrit word *tapas* is "heat." Make no mistake, grief is fiery; grief is work. And nobody else can do the work for us. I have frequently joked that I would like to have a yoga stand-in double – someone who would do a challenging physical yoga practice for me, and then I would just jump in for the "big pose," or the final resting pose, strong and fortified, glowing and restored. Sometimes I think I'd like an emotional stand-in double as well. That person could mindfully live through all my difficult and complicated life experiences and I would pop in for the highs and the happiness, looking fabulous, wise, and enlightened. It just doesn't work that way. Yoga is work. Life is work.

In this grieving process, we work not only to purify ourselves (*saucha*), but also to nourish ourselves. The practice of *tapas* combined with the practice of *ahimsa*, non-violence, means that we neither over-work nor under-work. We don't do too little or too much. It's what I call the Goldilocks approach: just right. And we practice self-care. Grieving people and those who help and support them need to practice self-care every day, renewing and replenishing our personal resources for the challenging work of grieving and loving those who mourn.

What restores your soul? Take at least five minutes each day to do it. Gradually build up a practice of self-care and notice how your spirit comes alive. Treat yourself at least as kindly as you would treat someone or something that you love and value.

What strengthens your will? Will-power is like a muscle; it needs to be exercised and conditioned. What life practices help you connect with your personal will-power and determination? As a means of strengthening self-restraint and impulse control, some yogis practice selective renunciation, or *tyaga*, in Sanskrit. *Tyaga* is the practice of giving something up in generosity or for the sake of fortifying personal will-power. *Tyaga* helps the practitioner let go of an object or habit in order to be free from attachment. For example, I really like coffee. I like the taste of it, I enjoy the aroma, I like something hot to drink in the morning, and I like to wrap my hands around a warm mug. Drinking coffee is part of the way I customarily begin the day. So as a *tyaga* practice, once in a while, I commit to a period of time during which I go without coffee. I don't give up coffee because it's "bad"; coffee isn't harmful to my health. I give up coffee because going without it is difficult for me. Drinking coffee is, for me, a strongly ingrained habit, and part of my morning routine. So giving up coffee from time to time helps me to strengthen my personal will power. As I do this *tyaga* practice, I exercise and flex my will-power "muscle," remember that my personal will-power is stronger than my habits, and relinquish attachment to coffee.

If I give up coffee, it doesn't necessarily benefit others. If I want to turn this particular *tyaga* practice into a practice of generosity, I could take an additional step of setting aside the money that I saved by not buying coffee and donating that money to charity.

Tapas: austerity and patience

The Sanskrit word *tapas* is often translated as "austerity." The Buddha said that enduring patience is the highest austerity. Yoga for grief and transition invites us to practice the austerity of patience. Neither yoga nor grief can be hurried. Processes such as these take as long as they take. Be patient, even with your own impatience. Courageously change the things you can change.

Questions about *tapas*

> ✿ *Fiery will-power and determination can arise within us around pursuits and ideas related to our true passions. What are your passions? About what do you feel and think passionately?*

> ✿ *Is there something you can let go of, something that is an impediment or obstacle to your healing? It might be a thought pattern or behavioral habit. Allow the intention to flow from your authentic being. What are you laying to rest today? Take small steps that can be accomplished successfully.*

❈ Is there something you might usher into your life that will bring you greater vitality, well-being, and wholeness? Again, allow this idea to come forth from the depths of your truth. What are you bringing to birth today? Find life-giving, life-affirming replacements for habits that are unproductive.

❈ Is there a specific goal you'd like to set for yourself? Something measurable and attainable?

❈ Think of a time in your life when you faced a significant challenge and conquered it. What personal resources did you engage? How did you order your life? Did you change your daily or weekly schedule to create time to accomplish your goal? Did you have a community of people supporting and encouraging you? What resources within you and around you are available now to support your growth through grief?

If you are working with a guide or a group, you might share your responses with one other person, or the group. Speaking our intention out loud makes it real in a non-scary way, and we can receive support from the people around us to make the changes that we intend.

4

Svadhyaya ~ Self-study

Practice reflection, contemplation, and observation.

Svadhyaya literally means "to recollect the Self," in other words, to remember who we are at the innermost core of our being. Because grief experiences often completely upset our sense of self and identity, turning the world as we formerly knew it upside down, they can actually direct us toward introspection and reflection.

Take time every day to reflect. Notice your life and your personal evolution. Practice witness consciousness. By this, I mean practice connecting with the part of yourself who is the observer, the unchanging one within you who can watch yourself, your thoughts, feelings, and behavior without judgment or criticism. The unchanging part of yourself is your true Self, your Being. Also observe and become familiar with that part of yourself that does change, your physical body, your thoughts, and your feelings. You are human. Humans feel and grieve and mourn and get angry. Feelings are neither bad or good; they are emotional energy. I sometimes use the image of climbing into an imaginary spaceship, and floating away from planet earth to watch myself – to watch my thoughts, my words, my actions, my feelings – and to make observations as though I were an objective yet compassionate observer. What might I notice about the patterns of my life, my thoughts, my words, and my actions?

Notice if your feelings propel you in one direction or another. Notice your responses or reactions to your feelings. Become acquainted with your own habits and ways of being, including your own emotional "triggers." Learn how to properly care for yourself, especially when you are hungry, angry, lonely, tired. (H.A.L.T.) Don't be afraid to ask for help or to accept help when it is offered, whether you need help with chores like plowing snow from the driveway and mowing the lawn, or you need a companion who can really listen to the pain of your heart.

After my husband died, I had many friends who called to offer their condolences and they often would say, "Let me know if you need help with anything." I would respond, "What can I put you down for? What sorts of things are you willing to do?" I kept a recipe box full of index cards in my kitchen and organized the box according to the types of chores and errands people had offered to perform. The following fall, a whole team of volunteers came to my home to help with the fall clean up. They washed windows, raked leaves, cleaned my garage, and brought good things to eat. After the chores were completed, we enjoyed a meal together. The giving and receiving became a single act of sharing our energy with each other, and we celebrated this exchange in our meal together.

Know your limits

In a spirit of non-violence, patience, and self-acceptance, come to know yourself and your limits. Many grieving persons and their caregivers find journaling to be a helpful and useful technique. Socrates said, "The unexamined life is not worth living." To that I add, "And the un-lived life is not worth examining." Self-study is different than self-analysis. Self-study is a practice in the context of a life fully lived. Come to know who you are, remembering your dignity, worth, and your own innate goodness. Wisely know the difference between the things you can courageously change and those things that are unchangeable, to which we have no choice but to surrender.

Questions for *svadyaya*

🕉 *Reflect on your own personality. Note any aspects of your personality that limit you, including self-limiting beliefs and stories that you've accumulated about yourself. Can these personality traits, beliefs, and stories be altered? If so, how?*

🕉 *What are you hoping to achieve in this life? What are your three most important goals, hopes, or desires? Where are you in terms of realizing your goals? Are you making daily choices that are consistent with what it is you truly desire in this life? If you are working with a group, you might share your reflections with others.*

❁ *In his book,* Structural Yoga Therapy, *Mukunda Stiles suggests spending some time with one or all of the following questions. Say the question to yourself several times and notice what arises in you. You may want to journal about your thoughts and feelings.*

> *Of what am I afraid?*
>
> *About what am I angry?*
>
> *To what am I holding on or clinging?*

5

Ishvara pranidhana ~ Practice humility and self-surrender

Ask for the serenity to accept the things you cannot change.

Ishvara in Sanskrit describes an all-pervading consciousness; *pranidhana* means "to surrender." Self-surrender is the practice of surrendering my humanity to a higher principle in the universe than my own small self. Some call it surrender to a Higher Power, Surrender to God, opening to Spirit or Presence, or living life with a big picture in mind. We must be brave enough to let go. If we are feeling burdened in this grieving process, we can begin to surrender the burdens when we remember and trust that there is someone to whom we can surrender them.

Ishvara pranidhana is a practice of tuning into the holiness and oneness of all life with confidence that all things in our life are working together for our good, even those things that are challenging and difficult. Tune into the light or Spirit within. The life force within is a gift, a blessing. You may not have a sense that this current experience – this death, or grief, or transition – is a blessing. That's okay. There's no benefit to candy-coating this current experience. It's okay to say, "I'm not liking this very much right now." That may be a practice in *satya*. As unpleasant as the current experience may be, we acknowledge the bigger picture, one that may be beyond our sight or imagination, tune in to the holiness of life, and acknowledge the gift of the life force within. We see our connectedness with one another, the universe, and a higher power or Spirit.

The French Jesuit philosopher and theologian, Pierre Teilhard de Chardin, is quoted as saying, "We are not human beings having a spiritual experience. We are spiritual beings having a human experience." *Ishvara pranidhana* honors the human person as innately spiritual, oriented toward the Presence that infuses all life. Surrender to this Presence invites us to be open to the possibility of receiving something greater than we have imagined for ourselves. We open to the gift of this day and this life, not as we rigidly plan, but by listening, opening, accepting and receiving. The love, strength, and support of others can help carry us through these transitions through the unknown and help us to experience Presence.

Albert Einstein said, "There are only two ways to live your life. One is as though nothing is a miracle. The other is as though everything is a miracle." The practice of *ishvara pranidhana* leads us to see everything, including our own, precious life, as a miracle.

Humility

The words human, humble, and humor are all derived from the same Latin root "*humus*," meaning earth. A human who is humble is literally close to the earth, or on the ground. The practice of humility and having a sense of humor is the practice of being fully human. Humility is not self-deprecation or self-defacement. Humility is authentically knowing who I am, being grounded in my true Self, not taking myself too seriously, and being able to kindly laugh at myself.

A salutation to remember that everything is a miracle

The Hindi word *namaste* is used in India to say hello and goodbye, excuse me, and thank you. The Indian people bring their hands to a prayer position in front of their hearts and bow to one another offering this greeting which translates something like, "The light in me honors the light in you," or "the eternal essence of me bows to your eternal essence." The word *namaste* reminds us to reverence the sacredness of every person.

An *ishvara pranidhana* practice for working with the mind, the emotions, and moving toward a higher perspective

The job of the mind is to think; it really never stops. We can't turn the mind off, but we can dial down certain parts of the mind, while turning up other aspects of the mind. For example, some parts of the mind are more concerned with taking in information, analyzing, communicating, or planning, while other parts of the brain are more attuned to experiencing the present moment and going with the flow of life. There is no one brain state that is superior to the others, though certain activities and responsibilities require us to be in the state of mind for the task at hand.

We do have control of the brain. We are not the victim of our own thoughts. If you appreciate visualization, you might imagine a dial on the front of the forehead which allows you to tune in to the mind channel that you need for a specific task.

We can also use this imaginary dial to help manage our emotions. Emotions aren't bad or good. Emotions are messengers of our needs, and help us to answer the question, "Are my needs being met?" Emotions can be useful, and if we want to bring our best selves forward, we need to learn to manage our emotions in the direction of positive energy. We need tools for accessing our inner resource.

Visualization practice for managing heavy or negative emotions

Begin by choosing a comfortable position. You may stand, sit, lie down, or take a walk while you do this practice. Allow yourself to be truly comfortable, and begin by bringing awareness to the sensations of your breath. Soften the muscles of the face, and relax into a state of conscious, present awareness. If it's useful, turn the imaginary dial on your forehead so that your mind is tuned to the "flow" channel.

Once you feel relaxed, imagine a difficult situation that has evoked sadness, agitation, anger, or frustration for you. It doesn't have to be something big and life-changing. Life is full of minor incidents that can be upsetting, depending on our state of mind. As you imagine this event or situation, notice the emotions. Notice and feel the physical sensations of the emotions. Notice where in your physical body these emotions create sensations of heaviness, dullness, constriction, or tension. Do you feel sensations in your face, throat, chest, belly, upper back, or lower back? Does breathing become quicker, more shallow, or more difficult as you feel the emotions?

Now name the emotions. Giving the emotions truthful names can be very powerful.

Accept the emotions. As a gesture of acceptance, hold out your hands, palms up, as though you are catching the emotions like little rain drops. How does it feel to catch the emotions in your hands?

Next, visualize climbing up a mountain and looking down on the emotions from a distance. See that your emotions are real, but they are not YOU; they are not your identity. You can leave them at the base of the mountain, and they will be there for you if you choose to pick them up again when you go back down.

Imagine going down and up the mountain. At the base of the mountain, take a moment to feel, acknowledge, and name the emotions. At the top of the mountain, look out and see the emotions from a higher perspective.

Next, pause at the top of the mountain, and as you gaze down to view the emotions, imagine someone else who is also suffering. All humans suffer. Imagine joining hands with someone else who is suffering, or with all of humanity, and offer and receive compassion. You might place both of your own hands over your own heart, and offer yourself a mini self-hug as a gesture of compassion.

Looking down from the mountaintop, you might ask, "What is the message of these emotions? Is there an insight or a higher purpose coming from this experience?" Be patient. It can sometimes take a long time – months, or even years – to receive the answer.

As Rainer Maria Rilke wrote in his *Letters to a Young Poet*, "Be patient toward all that is unsolved in your heart and try to love the questions themselves ... Do not seek the answers which cannot be given to you now because you would not be able to live them. And the point is to live everything. Live the questions now. Perhaps you will then gradually, without noticing it, live along some distant day into the answer."

Be gentle with yourself. This isn't a practice to evoke the "should haves," "could haves," or would haves." Silence the inner critic. Stop the self-destructive self-criticism. Your identity is so much greater than your wounds. "Be patient toward all that is unsolved in your heart."

Questions about *ishvara pranidhana*

- ❃ *Think of someone who seems to live life with the bigger picture in mind. How does this way of life affect their words, actions, and peace of mind?*

- ❃ *What does spirituality mean to you?*

- ❃ *How can you turn a mundane or necessary chore into a spiritual activity?*

- ❃ *Is there a spiritual practice or activity to which you feel particularly drawn at this time in your life because you believe that you would find it especially helpful and meaningful?*

Your Body, Your Heart, Your Mind, Yourself: *Chakras* and Healing Energy

*W*hen we are grieving, every aspect of our physiology can be affected by our experience of sorrow and trauma. In the early, raw stages of grief, we might feel as though we've been thrown completely off balance. Everything in the world might feel strange and unfamiliar, including the small universe of our own body and being. Even as we progress on the journey of grief, we might have experiences that trigger our wounds and throw us back to feeling baffled and discombobulated.

When one aspect of our being is distressed, the entire person suffers, for we are whole, even when we feel torn apart. The body, though it has many parts with diverse functions, is connected and is one, and the ancient yogis intuitively discerned a sense of the profound inter-connections and links between various parts of the human being and human body.

The ancient science of yoga anatomy identified a central channel or *nadi* (the name means "river"), which runs along the spine. This central channel, the *sushumna nadi*, was and is understood as a sort of super highway of energy moving the life force, or *prana*, along the spine and nourishing every cell of the body. Along the central channel, the yogis identified seven main energy centers, or *chakras*, in the body. A *chakra* is a wheel or vortex of energy in the subtle energy body of any living being. In the understanding of the ancient yogis, *chakras*, together with the *nadis*, make up the subtle energy body of all living beings. The seven *chakras* have some correlation to western science's understanding of the nervous system; modern physiological science shows that most of the seven *chakras* are located near the major nerve ganglia along the spinal column.

Exploring an understanding of the *chakra* system offers another way to understand ourselves. It may be useful to think of the *chakras* metaphorically or poetically rather than literally. If you are a scientist or an anatomist, you might be ready to dismiss this conversation about *chakras* because "they don't really exist." But, just to play yogi's advocate, are you familiar with the expression, "Butterflies in the stomach?" When you hear that expression, do you literally think of winged insects in your abdominal organ? Or do you relate to a light, fluttery sensation in the belly? If you were to say that you have butterflies in your stomach, I don't imagine that you literally have insects flying in your belly, but I do know, or can imagine, the physical, emotional, and energetic sensation of which you speak. Ayurvedic medicine and yogic science is very old, and still very useful, though the language system may seem completely foreign if you are just beginning.

According to this ancient science, the wheels of the *chakras* spin all along the spine in our bodies. Their energy is influenced by and in turn influences our physical, emotional, and spiritual health and balance. A little bit of knowledge about these energy centers and their functions can help us to recognize when we are not in balance and give us a richer understanding of and appreciation for the yoga techniques for wellness offered in this book.

Movements of the spine influence the nervous system

The physical practice of yoga *asana* or postures moves the spine in all directions – bending forwards, backwards, flexing, and extending, bending laterally to the left and right, and twisting across the body in both directions. These movements of the spine can release muscular tension, reduce fatigue, strengthen the muscles that help to hold the spine in healthy posture and, especially when combined with conscious breathing, awaken and manipulate the nervous system. In yogic thinking, this balances the *chakras* and promotes the flow of *prana*, our life force. Again, if this image is not useful to you, you may choose to understand yoga practices simply as exploring a diversity of movements in the spine and the physical body as a way to care for your body and brain. If you're interested in a simple exploration of the ancient yogis' intuitive wisdom about the human person, read on.

Seven *chakras* and five elements

Our experience of grief and loss can upset the harmony of the *chakras*, resulting in imbalance and disrupting the flow of prana. *Chakra* work can be helpful in restoring harmony and balance during times of grief.

Each of the seven main *chakras* is associated with a natural element – earth, water, fire, air, and space, or a particular element of human experience – sound, light, taste, sight, and thought. Like an internal rainbow, each *chakra* vibrates to a particular color – red, orange, yellow, green, turquoise blue, indigo, and violet. The ancient sages who divined the practice of yoga saw and experienced that what happened outside them in the universe of the created world also happened within them in the smaller but equally amazing universe of the human body and human experience.

The practice of yoga can become our own personal divining or discovery process. We can inquire deep within ourselves to discover the wellspring of vitality, health and wisdom in our own being. Because the *chakras* are related to elements and colors, simple methods for increasing their health and vitality include spending time in nature and the practice of color therapy. Notice if you gravitate toward certain colors during various phases of the grieving process, and notice how colors affect the flow of your emotions. Trust your intuition and bring color into your life that seems soothing, stimulating, or attractive to you according to your daily needs.

All of the *chakras* are connected to each other, just as everything in the body is connected. In yoga practice, we do not compartmentalize or isolate aspects of our being. You may notice, though, that throughout the first six *chakras* a pattern emerges in which the *chakras* alternately relate to practices of will or action and practices of grace or surrender. The first, third, and fifth *chakras* keep us connected to the energy of personal authority, willpower, courage, resolve, strength, truth and authenticity. The second, fourth, and sixth *chakras* align us with the energy of grace, flow, receptivity, and wisdom. The seventh *chakra* brings all these qualities into one, connecting and aligning us with love and the divine.

The first *chakra*: the root *chakra*

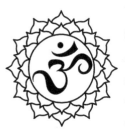

The first *chakra*, the *muladhara chakra*, is located at the base of the spine. *Muladhara* means root and foundation, so this *chakra* governs the roots and foundation of the body including all of the bones, muscles, and tissue of the legs and feet as well as the sits bones, tailbone, and organs of elimination. A healthy, balanced root *chakra* is essential to the health of the entire body and foundational to the balance of all the other *chakras*, so our discussion of the *chakras* begins with a more expansive conversation about the root *chakra*.

This first *chakra* is related to the element of earth and vibrates to the color red. Red is universally acknowledged as a power color. If you want to assert your authority, wear red – a red suit, tie, pants, shoes. Red makes a statement. Wearing red might make you feel more grounded and connected to you foundation. *Muladhara* represents survival, courage, authority, and a sense of being grounded. A healthy root *chakra* requires that all our basic needs of food, shelter, and clothing are met in a whole and balanced way. Experience of trauma and traumatic loss can make us feel un-earthed or unsafe, upset our sense of being grounded, shake our foundation, and cause us to feel worried or anxious about our livelihood and survival.

Balanced or blocked?

Symptoms of a root *chakra* that is blocked or out of balance might include:

- lower back pain
- digestive and elimination disorders
- hoarding or erratic spending
- overeating, under-eating, or dramatic changes in body weight
- feeling apprehensive or anxious
- feeling sluggish, lethargic or tired
- feeling disconnected, scattered, or disorganized
- being fearful about finances and worried about meeting your own basic needs

In our yoga for grief practice, **first *chakra* inquiry** includes questions:

- 🪷 *Do you trust and believe that your life will continue and that you will enjoy a good life even after this loss – whether the loss of a job, a relationship, or a beloved pet or person?*

- 🪷 *Did your beloved provide a sense of security and wellbeing for you?*

- 🪷 *Will all your basic needs be met? Will you have what you need for food and shelter?*

- 🪷 *What other concerns or questions arise as you navigate this journey of grief?*

In the grieving process, attention to our root *chakra* can give us some insight into the mystery of why we are feeling the way we do, and help us notice the ways in which this foundation of our being has been affected. If we can witness and notice any imbalances, then we can begin to move in the direction of a new state of wellness and wholeness.

Standing on our own two feet

A healthy root *chakra* is expressed first and foremost in faith and trust in the goodness of life. It is demonstrated in our body in the courage and confidence to stand on our own two feet, and in the ability to be grounded in our own, personal authority. But grief can literally knock us off our feet and have a physical impact on our bodies as well as mental and emotional effects.

Healthy feet are essential to a healthy body and skeletal structure. We might not give our feet and legs much attention unless they are causing pain and suffering that limits our capacity to ambulate through the world and accomplish the things we want and need to do. But in yoga, especially in these yoga for grief practices, we are attentive to building connection to strong, reliable, stable, grounded energy, and this attention and awareness begins at the soles of our feet.

There are 26 bones and 30 joints in the average human foot (some variations are present in the human population), so we see from its structure that the foot is designed for mobility and agility as well as stability. We can benefit the health of our root *chakra* by moving and stretching the feet before and after the practice of standing yoga poses, walking, and other standing and weight bearing activities.

The following pages share a simple practice for awakening the energy in your feet and connecting with your foundation, your root. Take off your shoes, and sit barefoot on the ground with your legs extended in front of you, or sit barefoot on a chair, taking a tall seat with the legs extended forward.

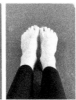

Breathe deeply and evenly, inhaling and exhaling through the nostrils.

1. As you exhale, flex the feet, drawing your toes toward your head, and spread the toes to your capacity. As you inhale, point and scrunch the toes to lengthen the tops of the feet. Repeat this six times or more.

2. Next, as you exhale, roll through the ankle so the soles of the feet face each other. As you inhale, roll through the ankle so the soles of the feet face each out and the toe nail sides of the feet face each other. Repeat this six times or more.

3. Now breathe deeply as you circle the foot and ankle through space in one direction, six times or more; then reverse the direction of the circles six times or more. After moving the joints of the feet, notice what you feel in the muscles of the legs. You might feel vibration all the way up to the base of the spine.

4. Finally, stand up, wiggle your toes, feel your feet, notice if you are standing more heavily on the right foot than the left, gather information about the alignment of your standing posture, and imagine sending breath down into the soles of your feet. You

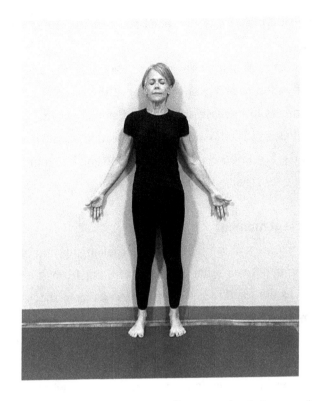

might stand with a wall at your back to experience the sensation of something solid literally "having your back."

You can practice this often. At the end of a day, take time to stretch and move your feet. Practice standing barefoot, outdoors on the earth when possible. While waiting in the cashier line at the grocery store or post office, notice your stance and imagine that you can breathe all the way down into the soles of your feet.

The physical practice of yoga and balancing the *muladhara chakra*

In our practice of standing yoga postures especially, we give great attention to active engagement of the muscles of the feet and legs to increase strength and stability in the lower extremities, which ultimately gives us freedom to move with ease and grace. Rooting in your foundation and breathing is a technique for staying present in the moment.

The present moment

Being truly present in the moment is challenging, and often even more difficult when we are suffering from grief or trauma, as the mind might try to protect us from shock and pain by escaping the present moment.

There's almost always something coming up in the future that we need to anticipate, but if the mind spins off and spends too much time imagining the future – "*what would happen if...*" – we may begin to experience feelings of anxiety. And many of our stories and memories of the past will bring us comfort and consolation, but if the mind spends too much time ruminating about the past, we might experience feelings of depression.

If we are perpetually being pulled away from the present moment, we will eventually be left feeling depleted, worn out, and out of touch with our true Self. Yoga practice helps us rehearse being present, using the breath, and anchoring the mind.

Here is a simple grounding practice

This practice is simple; remembering to do it can be challenging. When you are distressed or simply stressed, can you remember to ground yourself and breathe?

Bring awareness to all of your senses.

- ✧ Notice five things that you can see.
- ✧ Notice four things that you can physically touch and feel.
- ✧ Notice three different sounds you can hear. Notice if each sound has a beginning, a middle, and an ending.
- ✧ Notice any fragrances around you. Can you identify two distinct scents?
- ✧ Notice any taste in your mouth.

Being grounded in the present moment is a practice, so be patient and gentle with yourself. When we are grounded and present on our own two feet, we are standing in our own personal authority.

Be the author of your healing story

Our root chakra is connected to our personal authority, so someone who has a balanced, healthy root has authority, but is not authoritarian. The word "authority" shares the same root as the word "author," meaning to originate, to cause, to create, or to write a story. We are writing our own healing story. Each of us is our own best authority on our life, our experience, our body, and our emotions. As we become grounded in the authority of our physical, energetic, and emotional body, we discern how to heal ourselves.

A good yoga teacher has authority, but is not authoritarian. Using the metaphor of giving birth, a gifted yoga teacher, therapist, or counselor can serve the valuable role of midwife for our process of moving through grief, and each of us will give birth to our own transformed self in our own unique way. In the experiences and stories of our lives and in our internal, personal resources, we have been given priceless material for our own story of personal transformation.

Practices for a healthy root *chakra*

Restorative yoga postures are very nourishing to the root *chakra*, because they are practiced on the ground, close to the earth. Standing yoga poses awaken and balance the root *chakra*, and help us practice the attitude of being grounded in our authority. Working expressly with the feet, either in standing postures, stretching the feet, or massaging the feet with essential oils, is also very beneficial to the health of the feet and legs, thus supporting a healthy root *chakra*.

Other activities which are beneficial to the health of the root *chakra* include walking, especially walking in nature or walking barefoot in the dirt and grass, gardening (digging and working in the soil of the earth), and cooking good, clean, nutritious, natural food. The sense of smell is also associated with the first *chakra*, so cooking fragrant food and bringing aromatic flowers and elements of nature indoors can be nourishing and balancing for the root. Certain essential oils are also very therapeutic for this purpose.

Reflection questions for the root *chakra*

What's one thing you can do today, even a small thing...

> ✤ *to move in the direction of relieving anxiety about your future and your own well-being?*
> ✤ *to move in the direction of surrendering the burdens and heartaches of the past?*

Mula bandha: the root lock

One yogic technique often combined with the practice of *asana* (postures), *pranayama* (mindful manipulation of the breath), and meditation is the practice of *bandhas*. A *bandha* is a lock. As the *nadis* are energetic channels or rivers, the *bandhas* are like locks and dams on the river. The *bandhas* control and promote the flow of *prana* or life force through the entire spine. The practice of *bandhas* is a sophisticated practice for moving energy in an intentional way.

Mula bandha is the root lock, an intentional engagement of the muscles of the pelvic floor at the base of the spine. More precisely, the center of the pelvic floor, the perineum, lifts up and in the body to move prana into the central channel, the *sushumna nadi*. The practice of *mula bandha* strengthens and tones the muscles of the pelvic floor, so this practice is beneficial to the root *chakra* and the second *chakra*.

To experience the sensation of *mula bandha*, lie on your back on the floor, or on a bed. Allow the knees to fall open and the arms to rest along side the body. This pose is called *supta badha konasana*, or reclined bound angle pose. Press

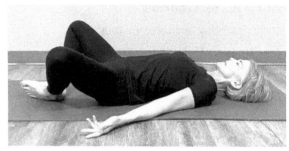

the soles of the feet together. You will feel the adductor muscles of the thighs engage. You will also feel the pelvic floor lift up and engage, and you will feel the abdominal wall lift up and in. The subtle lifting of the pelvic floor is the action of *mula bandha*. The action of the abdominal wall lifting up and in is called *uddiyana bandha*. Further description of *uddiyana bandha* follows in our discussion of the third *chakra*.

If you interlace the fingers and press your palms away, up and overhead, you might feel the abdominal wall lift up and in even more. Notice that you can continue to breathe deeply as you do this, though the shape of the body, which is

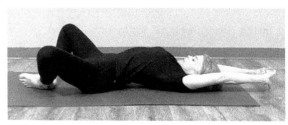

the container for the breath, has changed. You might feel the breath moving the ribs laterally away from each other more, and less inflation in the belly. Yoga techniques offer us many variations for the breath. There is no one correct way to breathe. If we want to work with our breath to heal ourselves and change our lives, there is no one, single correct way to do that.

The second *chakra*: the sacral *chakra*

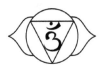 The second *chakra*, or *svadhisthana*, which relates to "sweetness," is located behind and below the navel. The energy of the second *chakra* governs the health and vitality of the organs of reproduction and the bones, muscles, and tissue of the hips, pelvis, and sacrum. Sacral *chakra* energy draws us towards partnership and is responsible for our feelings of emotional connection, pleasure, gratification, and creativity, so it's not surprising that the sacral *chakra* will be disturbed during periods of grieving, especially if we are grieving the loss of an intimate partner. The *svadhisthana chakra* is associated with the element of water, including our own tears, and vibrates to the color orange.

Just a couple of months after Chad died, I remember walking past a small boutique in my neighborhood and seeing bright orange linen overalls on the mannequin in the window. I don't think I had ever owned a piece of orange clothing before in my life, but I had to have those overalls. I bought them and wore them so much that summer that the color faded from washing and exposure to the sun. The orange color expressed the confidence, joy, and enthusiasm that I wanted to feel but couldn't quite summons from within myself because I was overwhelmed by grief.

While the first *chakra* is concerned with stability and foundation, the second *chakra* is concerned with fluidity, sensuality, inspiration, creativity, family, and playfulness. In addition to yoga postures that open the hips, the practice of yoga postures combined with intentional breathing patterns (vinyasa yoga), dancing, making music, and other playful, flowing movement can help bring balance to the second *chakra*. Think of the soothing, rhythmic rocking of a boat on the water. This is second *chakra* energy. It is spontaneous and free.

Trauma and grief upset the rhythm and flow of our lives. Restoring the flow and nourishing the health of the second *chakra* is a practice of grace and receptivity. Dancing, swimming, playful, spontaneous activity, breath-based yoga exercises and any creative endeavors are all very nourishing for the second *chakra*, as are meaningful human interaction and emotionally satisfying relationships.

List all of the ways you enjoy expressing your creativity, both big and small. It can be anything – drawing, painting, dancing, writing, cooking, singing, playing an instrument – or something you do in your profession like public speaking, teaching, coding, leading, healing. How are you creative?

Creative endeavors connect us to our own unique life force and help us remember that we are truly alive.

❋ *Do you catch yourself feeling a sense of guilt when you are enjoying life, as though somehow you are betraying the memory of a loved one who can no longer experience these sensations or pleasures? What compassionate words of encouragement can you offer yourself to affirm the goodness of your own life and the importance of enjoying it?*

❋ *Are you struggling to forgive yourself for things you wish you had or had not said or done? Are you struggling to forgive someone else? How can you see this situation in the most loving way possible? What would you say to a dear friend or beloved child who was suffering in a similar way?*

❋ *As a flow activity, making music or listening to music can be nourishing and healing for the second chakra. Is there a particular piece of music that helps you connect to the memory of your loved one or an important time or event together? The music might elicit an emotional response. Can you give yourself permission to cry, or laugh or dance?*

❋ *In yoga for grief, we work to be the witness, not the judge, off our emotions. What beliefs do you hold about crying? Do you let yourself cry when you need to, or do you believe that crying makes you "weak?"*

The third *chakra*: the solar plexus

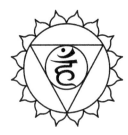

The third *chakra*, the *manipura chakra*, is located in the solar plexus, the sun center or seat of fire of the body. *Manipura* is related to the element of fire. It includes the muscles of the abdomen and mid-back. The energy of the third *chakra* governs the function of the digestive system, the liver, the pancreas, and the gallbladder. Here in the belly are located more nerve endings than in the brain. This is the body's center of personal willpower and emotional intelligence, hence expressions like "gut instinct," "gut sense," and I've got "guts"; I'm "gutsy." When the third *chakra* is healthy and balanced, we know who we are and we have a clear sense of purpose in our lives.

The sudden or traumatic loss of a loved one or a relationship, a home or a job can feel like a sucker punch to the gut; grief can be "gut wrenching." My son's comment that he felt like he had a "big hole in his tummy" after my husband died was an insightful observation on his part of the way that grief showed up in his body.

The third *chakra* governs personal willpower, determination, courage, and valiance. It is our core, our center of authenticity. When we are grieving we might feel overwhelmed by a sense of powerlessness against the great mysteries of life and death and the unfairness of it all. Life isn't fair. As I used to tell my son, "The fair comes once a year, and this isn't it." The paradox of power is that we are always both powerful and powerless. Even when life is "unfair," we have power to make choices and to chose our response to our circumstances.

🏵 *What does "power" mean to you?*

🏵 *When and where in your life have you felt powerful?*

🏵 *How do you feel powerful at this time?*

🏵 *When and where in your life have you felt powerless?*

🏵 *How do you feel powerless at this time?*

A personal story of valiance and resilience

I consider myself both a trauma survivor and a grief survivor. I prefer the term "survivor" to the word "victim" because "survivor" implies valiance and resilience.

I've had multiple experiences of trauma in my life. As I mentioned briefly in my personal loss inventory, I grew up with a brother who had manic-depressive bipolar disorder. That meant that, among other disruptions to our family's life, when he was having a psychotic episode, our home could get wildly chaotic and I didn't always feel safe.

In a more recent experience of trauma from my adult life, I was abused by a boss at my primary place of employment. Through that prolonged traumatic experience, I never referred to myself as his "victim." Rather, I considered myself the "target" of his abuse. I believed that I could not allow myself to succumb to a victim mentality if I wanted to survive and ultimately outlast him.

- ❁ *What makes you feel angry?*
- ❁ *What makes you feel afraid?*
- ❁ *What is important or sacred to you?*
- ❁ *What gives you a sense of purpose?*

This is third *chakra* inquiry. Being truthful about these third *chakra* emotions can set us free to move through them and use the energy of the emotions, rather than deny them. Anger is not inherently evil; anger is a call to action. A balanced third *chakra* allows us to take right action, rather than simply react, when we feel angry.

When my abusive boss was creating a hostile work environment for me, I felt both anger and fear; I felt angry about the injustice of the situation and I felt afraid for my livelihood and wellbeing. Anger gave me the energy I needed to protest the injustice, to take a stand against the abuse, to take appropriate action against the perpetrator, to hold my ground, and to finally outlast him, even when I felt afraid.

A gut feeling is actually every cell
in your body making a decision."
~ Deepak Chopra

Cultivating core traits for a healthy third *chakra*

I have cultivated many personal qualities over my lifetime that have given me the endurance to outlast the hostile, abusive, offensive behavior of my boss:

- ❀ *I know who I am, I believe in my own innate goodness.*
- ❀ *I have self-knowledge and self-understanding, and I work to practice self-compassion.*

Regarding my work, which I experience as a calling or vocation:

- ❀ *I am confident that the work I do is important to the people I serve.*
- ❀ *I have a strong sense of purpose in my job, and I have forged authentic human connection with the people who benefit from my work.*

My dedication, perseverance, and sense of purpose helped me to survive that horrible job-related situation.

The healing power of community

Experiences of trauma and grief can trigger emotions that would disconnect us from the "core" of our own true nature. Having people in our lives who support the journey of reconnection promote our healing process. Though my experience of abuse by my boss, I was very fortunate to have a few trustworthy people in my life who truly saw, heard, and understood me, who validated the reality of the hostile conditions of my work environment, who valued and respected me, who affirmed my goodness, and who trusted my authentic identity and character.

Research has linked social isolation and loneliness to higher risks for a variety of physical and mental conditions. One popular tactic of abusers is to try to isolate their targets from people who would offer support, to make the target believe that she is alone or, worse yet, crazy. Despite his efforts, my abuser was unsuccessful in isolating me. My work of healing from trauma and grief was supported by a select community of individuals who encouraged me to stand powerfully and courageously in my own authentic Self.

Laughter

The third *chakra* is also a center of humor. ***When and where do you experience laughter and a sense of playfulness or recreation?*** Think of a good belly laugh. Few things are more beneficial to our sense of vitality and well-being than laughter that comes from deep in our core, but when we are grieving, we might experience a lack of laughter and fun in our lives. When the core *chakra* is in balance, we have a steady sense of confidence, self-worth, and humor. We are at ease in our true identity. A sense of humor and humility are essential in the transformational work of yoga.

This work is difficult. It requires great gentleness and patience. It can sometimes feel heavy, so we look for the qualities of lightness and radiance. Think of the color yellow, the color to which the *manipura chakra* vibrates. Yellow represents the lightness of third *chakra* energy. Yoga *asana*, postures, when practiced properly, require strength and stability in the center of the body, as well as good, easy space that is without tension and gripping.

Rest

A healthy third *chakra* needs time to rest and digest. We need time and rest to digest our food, we need time and rest to digest our life, we need time and rest to digest our experiences, joyful and sorrowful, and we need time and rest to process our emotions.

Resting in a supported restorative pose that opens the belly helps to clear the digestive system and cleanse the nervous system. A supported reclined pose when practiced with sufficient props to support the whole spine, including the low back and neck, is an excellent pose for this purpose.

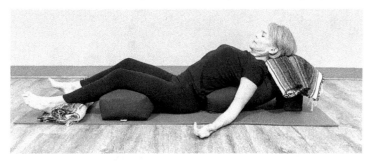

"We work very hard in our lives, and while we may sleep, we rarely take time to rest. Restorative yoga poses help us learn to relax and rest deeply and completely."
~Judith Hanson Lasater

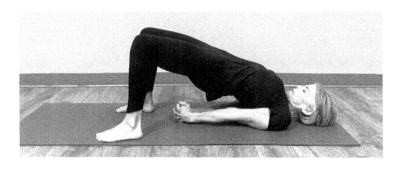

Uddiyana bandha is the abdominal lock. Uddiyana literally means "flying up," and suggests the upward lifting energy of this bandha which is practiced by lifting the navel up and in toward the spine. The abdominal lock brings strength and stability to the core body, awakens the energy at the manipura chakra and, in connection with mula bandha, is lightly engaged in many yoga postures. One safe and accessible ways to learn uddiyana bandha is to practice it in bridge pose. We will further explore that in the practice portion of this book.

Manipura Chakra Reflection questions

🪷 Grief is hard work. Do you trust yourself and believe that you're capable of doing hard things? What is an example of something difficult that you've done or accomplished in your life? What personal qualities and resources did you employ to do it?

❀ What's one small difficult thing you can do today to practice trusting and exercising your own power? (Sometimes asking for help or assistance is a difficult thing, and doing it might make you feel empowered.)

❀ Do you believe that you have power to make small but significant choices? For example:

    ❀ What time will you get up in the morning?

    ❀ How will you begin your day? Meditation, exercise, journaling, prayer, breakfast? How will you conclude each day? What time will you choose to go to bed?

    ❀ Are there end of the day rituals – disconnecting from electronics and devices, meditation, prayer, journaling, or restorative yoga – that you will choose to reduce muscular tension and fatigue and increase your ability to rest well?

❀ Are you confident in your own decision making abilities? Do you have advisors you trust to help you make important decisions?

❀ Can you give yourself permission to assert your boundaries with respect and clarity?

❀ Patience requires tremendous will power, courage, and discipline. In what ways are you demonstrating patience and discipline in this grieving process?

❀ Do you allow yourself to feel all your emotions, including anger or fear? What message do you think your emotions are communicating to you today?

The fourth *chakra*: the heart

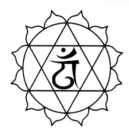 The fourth *chakra*, *anahata*, is located in the center of the chest, the energetic region of the heart. It governs the vital organs of the lungs, the heart, and the circulatory system and includes the bones, muscles, and tissue of the area around the sternum, the rib cage, the shoulders and upper back, the arms, the hands, and the breasts. Related to the element of space and vibrating to the color green or pink, when in balance, the heart is filled with compassion, devotion, acceptance, and faith. We might naturally think that heart *chakra* would be most affected by experiences of grief, because our heart has indeed been broken by loss. We have begun our work at the root, working from the ground up, because a truly open, balanced, and free heart chakra will need the stability, grace, and strength of the lower three *chakras* as a foundation of support.

The name of the *chakra*, *anahata*, means "unstruck." One interpretation of the name *anahata* is that there is, within the heart, a harp-like instrument that plays beautiful music without need of someone to pluck the strings. Without striking the instrument, the music plays on. Nourishing the fourth *chakra* helps us re-connect with our own life's music, the beautiful song or composition that is our unique life. There may be parts of the song that are slow, sad laments, and others that are more joyful, but the music is beautiful and uniquely ours.

Another interpretation of the name *anahata* is unblemished, unspoiled, or unhurt, implying that within the center of our own heart is a sanctuary that is un-touched by our stories of pain or tragedy. Our identity is so much more than our story or biography. Beneath our smaller personal stories of brokenness and pain lies a great true story of steadiness, sureness, resilience, and tranquility, a wellspring of wholeness and boundless unconditional love. Meister Eckhart, the 14th-century German mystic, expressed this idea when he wrote, "There is a place in the soul that neither time nor space nor no created thing can touch." In other words, there is a place in each of us, an inner sanctuary, where we have never been wounded, where there is steadiness, tranquility and connection to Spirit, Presence, Source, or a Higher Power. The practice of yoga, meditation, and contemplation offers the opportunity to visit this inner sanctuary and connect with Spirit or Source. Reading poetry, studying spiritual texts, singing and listening to inspired songs, and prayer, whether personal or with a faith community, can support your journey toward healing a broken heart and experiencing the peace and serenity of your inner sanctuary.

According to ancient eastern medicine, grief is stored in the lungs. In yoga for grief, we practice postures and *pranayama* (breath work) to open the heart center in a supportive way and tenderly move the energy of grief out of the heart and lungs, making space to visit the inner sanctuary.

Forgiveness

When we think about "opening" the energetic center of the heart, we might think first of the front side, but what about the back side of the heart center? The back side of the body in general, and the back side of the heart center in particular, can represent all that is behind us – the past. The past is the past; it cannot be changed. ***"Letting go of all hope of having had a better past,"*** may be the most useful definition of forgiveness that I have found. Forgiving people who have hurt us does not necessarily exonerate them – they may or may not deserve exoneration – but it does set us free of the burdens of bitterness and resentment. Maybe we need to forgive ourselves, too. If we made mistakes in the past, is it possible that we did the best we could with the information that we had at the time?

Warrior II

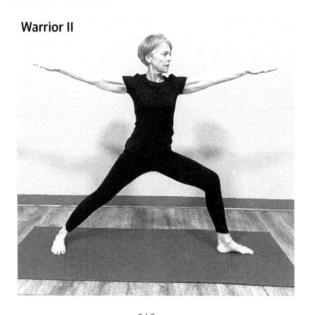

In the Warrior II sequence in the practice portion of this book, we embody the integration of the energy of the lower four *chakras*. In Warrior II we stand on our own two feet – stable, agile, and flexible – ready to move powerfully into the future. The center of the body is strong and not collapsed. We fearlessly gaze over the fingertips of the front hand into the mysterious unknown keeping an open heart, even when things get stressful or difficult. We are open to grace, connected with will and power, and practicing giving and receiving, breath by breath. All sides of the energetic center of the heart – front, back, left and right, are open and free.

Practice and reflection

Find a comfortable seated or reclined position. Place one hand over the center of your chest, and press your other hand on top of it. Breathe deeply into the space beneath your hands.

- 🪷 *Do you feel comforted, soothed, loved? What positive practices can you incorporate into your life to show yourself more compassion, empathy, and self-acceptance?*
- 🪷 *Describe two or three moments in your life when you felt deeply loved.*
- 🪷 *Describe two or three moments in your life when you felt deep love for another being.*
- 🪷 *How is this experience of love available to you now, even as you grieve?*

As you write or speak about these moments, notice sensations of warmth, vibrations of peacefulness and ease in your body, and any changes in the expressions of your face. When we are grieving, prayer can be a valuable part of our healing journey, and knowing that others are praying for us can strengthen us and lift us up as we move forward in our process.

- ❀ What, if any, spiritual or religious practices have been a valuable part of your life in the past?
- ❀ Are there daily, weekly, or seasonal rituals and ceremonies that you find meaningful and useful that you want to incorporate into your life at this time?

Religious and spiritual practice can be a way of giving back, metaphorically or literally linking hands with others who are on the human journey. Many faith communities offer opportunities to serve the common good. Selfless service not only benefits others; it helps us know that we are not alone.

- ❀ Is there a spiritual practice, individual or communal, that you could include in your life at this time to support your healing and inspire your hope?
- ❀ Is there a practice of service that you feel inclined to incorporate into your life at this time?

The fifth *chakra*: the throat

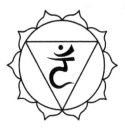

The *vissudha chakra* is physically located in the mouth, neck, jaw, and throat and includes the organs of the ears and throat, the thyroid and parathyroid. This *chakra* is known as the purification center, and governs the physical, emotional, and energetic function of communication. When the *vissudha chakra* is healthy and balanced, we connect with higher knowledge and speak our truth with confidence and kindness. We find our voice, and creativity and self-expression flourish.

Vissudha chakra disturbances are not uncommon during periods of grief. Feeling "all choked up," experiencing pain in the neck and shoulders, and even a throat that feels raw and sore are not uncommon when grieving.

Simple and frequent movement of the neck and shoulders can stimulate a stagnant throat chakra. Keeping the neck warm and massaging your own neck and throat and will soothe a depleted throat chakra, as will drinking lots of clean, clear water.

> "Listen, are you breathing just a little,
> and calling it a life? ...
> Oxygen.
> Everything needs it:
> bone, muscles, and even,
> while it calls the earth its home, the soul."
> **~ Mary Oliver**

Chanting and singing stimulate the throat chakra, as do other artistic forms of self-expression. Be sure to warm up the voice properly before singing, public speaking, or any situation that requires projection of the voice. The *vissudha* is related to the element of air or sound and vibrates to the color turquoise blue.

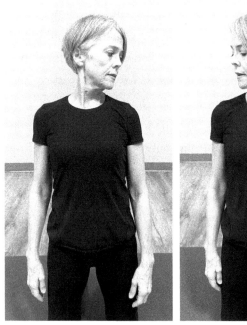

Try this simple sequence of extending, flexing, and twisting the neck. Find a comfortable standing or seated position. Breathe deeply, and slowly rotate the face to the right and left six to 20 times, or more. Avoid movement that creates crackling and popping sounds. Then pause.

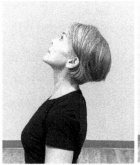 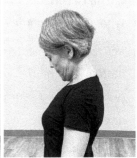

Next, extend and flex the neck, inhaling to look up and exhaling to lower the chin towards the chest. Again, repeat this action six to 20 times or more. When you extend the neck to look up, be sure you can swallow. If you're unable to swallow, you've overextended the throat.

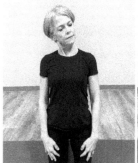 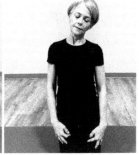

Now, breathe deeply and flex the neck to the left and the right, tilting your ear toward your shoulder. Move slowly and gently six to 20 times or more in each direction. These actions should not create any pain or suffering. Work within your own healthy range of motion to release tension in the neck and shoulders.

Vissudha *chakra* reflection:

- ❁ *What is your favorite form of self-expression?*

- ❁ *Reflect on this statement: "My voice and my words matter." List all the ways in which this is true. How are you finding your voice in new ways through this grieving process?*

- ❁ *In this grieving process, are there any situations in which you feel like you are faking or forcing yourself to be someone or something you're not? How do you feel when that happens?*

- ❁ *Write about a time when you spoke your truth and felt valued and respected and as though you had genuinely been heard. How did this make you feel?*

- ❁ *It can be difficult to find words to speak about our own grieving experience, and it can be challenging to adequately express our support for someone else who is grieving. That's okay; silence and presence are also powerful methods of communication. We can pretend to care, but we cannot pretend to show up.*

Jalandhara bandha, the throat lock

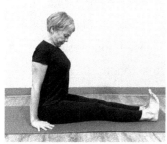

The practice of *jalandhara bandha*, the throat lock, is a nourishing practice for the *vissudha chakra*. In *jalandhara bandha*, the sternum lifts toward the chin, creating length in the entire spine, and the chin drops to the chest.

Jalandhara bandha spontaneously occurs in some yoga poses such as bridge pose (*setu bandha sarvangasana* in Sanskrit), plow pose (*halasana*), and supported shoulder stand (*salamba sarvangasana* and its variations). When we lift the chin away from the chest releasing the *bandha*, a fresh flow of blood and lymph circulates in the region of the throat, supporting the health of

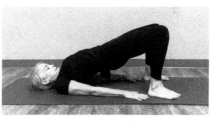

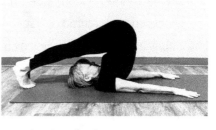

the endocrine system and strengthening the immune system. When *jalandhara bandha* is practiced in combination with *mula bandha* and *uddiyana bandha*, this is called *maha bandha*, the great lock. This is a technique for regulating the flow of energy in the spine.

The sixth *chakra*: the third eye

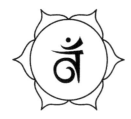

The *ajna chakra* or command *chakra* is located in the mid-brain, behind the center of the forehead and above the soft palate of the mouth. It governs the pineal gland, a light sensitive gland producing melatonin, the hormone which regulates sleeping and waking up. The third eye is related to the element of light and governs vision, insight, and intuition. In many yoga postures we practice *drishti*, or specific gazing points, to nourish and strengthen the muscles around the tiny ball and socket joint that is the eye. *Drishti* also helps to bring the mind to one pointed stillness, enlightening and strengthening the inward eye. The third eye *chakra* is your body's energy center for intuition, imagination, mental strength, inner wisdom, open-mindedness, and clarity. When we experience trauma or tragedy, life might seem completely cloudy and unclear, and we may find it difficult to trust our own intuition and inner wisdom.

The physical eyes and the muscles surrounding them hold and express emotion. We connect with other humans through eye contact and facial expression. When we are sad or afraid, tears may spontaneously flow from our eyes. During times of grief and stress, whether we express our emotions or repress our emotions, we may feel physical sensations of strain and fatigue in the eyes, the facial muscles around them, and the mid-brain.

In yogic meditation, sets of exercises are presented to soothe and restore the eyes, and to improve concentration and outward and inward sight. One such technique is the practice of *trataka*, a practice of focusing the gaze on a candle, flower, or other beautiful object to relax the eyes and even induce cleansing tears.

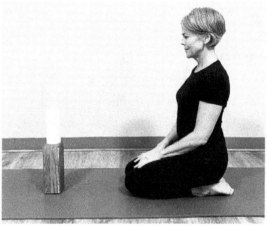

Try this method of *trataka*: Light a candle. Sit in a comfortable position where you can see it at eye level and at arm's length. Relax all eighty muscles of the face. Stare steadily at the dark part in the center of the flame until you can no longer maintain the gaze or until you release tears. Then close your eyes and focus on the image of the flame that remains in your mind's eye. When the image fades, rub your hands together to create some heat. Cup your warm hands around the eyes to soothe and comfort your eyes. Don't press your palms directly into your eyes; press the heel of the hands into the cheek bones and the ball mounts of the fingers into the brow bones. As you inhale, slowly open your eyes into the darkness of your hands. Stare into the darkness and be open to the unknown. Slowly release your hands away, allowing the eyes to adjust to the light of the room. Open your eyes and repeat the exercise. This exercise can be practiced with a beautiful or venerable object in place of a candle. The technique remains the same.

Eye exercises

If your daily work routine requires large amounts of "screen time," take regular breaks throughout the day to exercise your eyes. Look far away from your computer screen, then close your eyes. Rub your hands together until they're warm.

Cup your warm hands over your closed eyes. Don't press your palms directly into your eyes but press the heel of the hands into the cheek bones and the ball mounts of the fingers into the brow bones. As you inhale, blink your eyes open into the darkness of your hands, and as you exhale, close your eyes, lubricating them with your tears. Repeat this several times before taking your hands away from your eyes. Notice how your eyes feel. Blink and breathe.

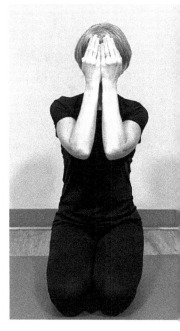

Distance gazing

Another stress reliever and strengthener for your eyes is the practice of distance gazing. Direct your gaze toward a distant object. If you're indoors, look out a window, if possible. Focus on the object as clearly and restfully as possible, staying relaxed in the muscles of the eyes and face. Take deep breaths. Then slowly shift your gaze to another distant object. Continue letting your eyes drift about the world around you, momentarily pausing at objects at varying distances away from you, and "drinking in" the images you see. If you spy something particularly pleasing, smile, enjoy the vision, and relax your mind. Imagine your eyes are being nourished and renewed in this practice, and give thanks for your strong, healthy eyes.

Reflection questions

- 🏵 *In what areas of your life do you believe you have a strong sense of clarity?*
- 🏵 *In what areas do you sense confusion or a lack of clarity?*
- 🏵 *Think of a time in your life when you showed incredible mental strength. What thoughts, beliefs, emotions, and personal qualities allowed you to hold onto this mental strength, even when it was difficult?*
- 🏵 *How do you most often experience your intuition? Does it come in the form of a gut feeling, a small, still voice inside you, signs or synchronicities, or something else?*

The seventh *chakra*: the crown

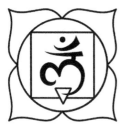 The physical description of the *sahasrara chakra* is usually the pituitary gland. This *chakra* is located about four fingers above the crown of the head. The name "*sahasrara*" means thousand, and refers to the thousand petaled lotus flower and its nectar. The crown *chakra* integrates the respective qualities and rainbow colors of all the *chakras*.

Representing the sweet nectar of understanding, expanded consciousness, and universal principles of connection to mystery and spirit, when the crown *chakra* is in balance we experience bliss, contentment, self-knowledge, the humility of self-emptiness, and a sense of connection to others and the divine.

Connection to others and connection to the Divine Presence, Source, or Spirit – however we choose to name it – is powerful medicine on the healing journey of grief. I've had a life-long connection to a faith community, and after Chad died, this became a critical connection for support in my healing journey of grief. In this community, I had a friend and spiritual director who was my trusted companion in the grieving process. I remember saying to her one day, through tears of frustration, "Everyone tells me that I'm so strong. I'm tired of being strong." She wisely responded, "Maybe you need to learn to be weak."

The paradox is that, when we are connected to Source or Spirit, in our weakness, we are strong. Strength is made perfect in surrender.

The crown *chakra* is related to the element of thought and vibrates to the color violet or white. Postures which place the crown of the head on the earth and stack the seven *chakras* in alignment serve the development of vitality in the crown *chakra*. Practices of prayer, chanting, and meditation nourish this *chakra*.

Reflection questions

- *What (or who) is Sacred, or Spirit, or God for you? What is your relationship with a higher power? How is that relationship evolving through this grieving process?*
- *What does it mean to you to surrender to a higher power? In what ways is this easy or difficult for you?*
- *Surrendering to a higher power can be difficult because it may feel like giving up personal control and losing a sense of personal power. However, in what ways does surrendering actually give you a greater sense of personal power?*
- *What are three ways you can practice surrendering in your daily life?*
- *Do you have a favorite prayer or spiritual song or chant? How might you incorporate it into your practice of yoga for grief?*

To begin a simple meditation practice, four things are necessary:

1. A quiet place.
2. An internal or external object on which to focus attention, the breath itself or a candle, flower, or sacred object for directing the gaze and mind.
3. An attitude of acceptance and receptivity.
4. A comfortable position, reclined, seated, standing or walking.

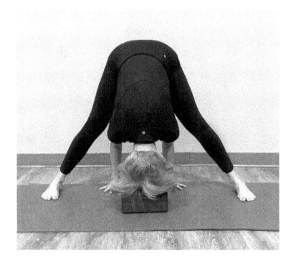

As a physical practice to stimulate the crown chakra, you might try this wide stance forward fold with a block under the crown of the head.

1% Theory, 99% Practice

Yoga "Guruji" Sri K. Pattabhi Jois taught that yoga is "99% practice and 1% theory." So, let's practice. "Practice and all is coming." Please tailor this practice of *Yoga for Grief, Transition, and Loss* to your needs and your life. You are your own best personal authority on the practices that benefit your healing process. *Pranayama* (yogic breathing), *asana* (the practice of postures), chanting, prayer, *mudra*, meditation, and ritual can all be elements of a yoga practice. Each individual can choose methods that are personally relevant and healing. Daily practice is the most effective method. Even five minutes each day of practicing one technique that feels meaningful to you will bring positive results.

If you are practicing these exercises on your own, you might record yourself narrating a guided sequence and play the recording to support your practice. If you are practicing with a group, you might play the recording for the group or have a companion or teacher read this narrative or other words that are authentic for your group. When you have more time, practice 20 minutes or longer.

Satsanga – practicing the healing power of community

In Sanskrit, the word *sat* means true and *sanga* is company, so *satsanga* is the practice of sitting in company with persons who listen to, talk about, and assimilate the highest truth. If you are doing this practice with a group, you may want to sit in a circle and begin by mutually agreeing on ground rules for confidentiality, mutual consideration, and support. All persons in the group are invited to experience the work in the way that is most authentic and beneficial to them. Let all those present agree to honor each individual in the group. If there are other agreements that the members of the group need in order to feel safe and respected, this is a time to establish those agreements. The group may want to put their covenant in writing. Next, create some kind of opening ritual such as asking each member of the group to share a word or phrase or sentence that describes how they are feeling, or have a deck of cards with words, phrases or sentences that support themes of healing and personal power and ask each person to draw a card and read it. Give each member of the group an opportunity to find his or her own personal voice. Once the group feels gathered and united, let each person settle into their own space for practice.

The progression of the practice sequence

The overall arch of the sequence of practices that I am offering here begins with reclined postures combined with breathing and visualization. Either of the reclined postures with visualization could be a complete practice in their own right. From a reclined position, I have then included a dynamic bridge sequence as a gentle spinal warm-up before progressing to standing poses.

In the interest of keeping the practice highly accessible, I recommend practicing standing postures first before practicing postures seated on the ground. Healthy alignment of the spine, hips, and knees is generally more accessible for the beginner in standing poses than in seated postures. All of the standing and seated poses can be supported by the use of props and can be modified to be practiced seated on a chair.

Breathing

On a purely physiological level, breath is important for several reasons. Breathing is the means by which we supply our bodies with oxygen, which is essential for the health of the brain, the nervous system, the glands, and the internal organs. Oxygen is essential to our well-being and survival; without it, we would die within a few minutes. Breathing is also a primary means of eliminating waste products and toxins from the body for cleansing and detoxification.

Our breath is also like a barometer for our life, our energy, and our yoga practice; it can reveal how we are feeling. When we are happy, content, or relaxed, our breath tends to be slow and deep. When we are agitated or unhappy, it becomes fast, shallow or completely stops. Breathing is both involuntary and voluntary, so we can change the pace and rhythm of our breath to alter our mood and consciousness. What we do with our breath affects our mind, our body, our nervous system, and our life. It's interesting that in many languages the word for breath can also be translated as Spirit.

A word about the autonomic nervous system

The autonomic or involuntary nervous system is classically divided into two subsystems, the sympathetic nervous system and the parasympathetic nervous system. The parasympathetic nervous system governs the body's rest and digest mode. Its action is complementary to that of the sympathetic nervous system. The sympathetic nervous system is constantly active at a basic level to maintain a stable, consistent environment in the body. The sympathetic nervous system helps us relate to and interpret stimuli from the world around us. When we perceive that we are in danger or under stress, the sympathetic nervous system mobilizes the body's fight, flight, or freeze response. Often, after traumatic life experiences, the sympathetic nervous system remains in "overdrive."

Frequently in yoga practice, our first task is to de-stress and to dial down the fight, flight, or freeze response, balancing and soothing the nervous system. One highly accessible method of doing this is by directing our awareness to the sensations of our breath and creating a breathing pattern that is slow, smooth, steady, deep and even. In this yoga for grief practice, we use mindful yogic breathing combined with yoga postures and simple methods of conscious relaxation and meditation.

Yogic breathing or *pranayama*

Prana is the Sanskrit word for life-force, or vital energy. *Yama* is a Sanskrit word meaning restraint. Does *pranayama* mean the restraint of our vital energy, or is the word a contraction for *prana-ayama*, meaning breath that is without restraint? The answer is yes. In yoga practice, *pranayama* is the practice of deliberate and mindful breathing, based on the belief that prana, the Spirit, or vital life force, is held within the breath. Deepening awareness and control over our breathing helps to unite the conscious with the unconscious mind.

In all yoga practice, we start where we are. When working with the breath, we begin by practicing simple self-study, and taking inventory of the current condition of the breath and the emotional, energetic body. We can do this from any comfortable position – standing, seated, reclined, or even walking – while taking a moment to witness the following:

- 🪷 *Am I breathing through my nose or mouth?*
- 🪷 *Am I breathing predominantly through one nostril?*
- 🪷 *When the breath enters the body, where do I feel shape change in the cavities of my body?*
- 🪷 *Does my chest, rib cage, and belly move freely to receive the breath?*

We are gathering information, not passing judgment. This is a practice in self-observation in a spirit of self-acceptance. When the attention is focused on the breath, notice the quality of the mind.

Notice if the simple act of bringing awareness to the breath caused you to breathe more slowly and deeply. This is often the case. (Notice if your breath is changing even as you read or hear these words.) Gradually invite the breath to enter and exit through the nose, if your sinuses allow this. As you exhale fully through the nose and inhale through the nose, allow the breath to slow down and becomes deeper. If you're exhaling to a count of three or four, see if you can inhale to a comparable count. If you want to play with precision in this practice, you can work with a metronome. Eventually, slowing the breath to about six breaths per minute (a five-second inhalation and a five-second exhalation) will have a quieting effect for the nervous system. Keep in mind, though, that any straining of the breath will be counterproductive. This practice is not aimed toward a goal of perfection or precision; rather, the purpose is to liberate ourselves from stress and tension and begin to let go of some of the burdens and restraints of the mind and body.

Change your breath to change your thoughts; change your thoughts to change your life

Ancient yogic wisdom teaches that when we change our breath, we change our experience of and response to our emotions and also change the patterns and habits of our mind. When we change our mind, we change our perspective and our ability to respond to the circumstances of our life. In *Yoga for Grief, Transition, and Loss* we work with our breath to cultivate this breath-brain connection, to work with our life in its current condition, one breath at a time.

The experience and wisdom of our life journey is in every cell of our body. When we anchor ourselves in our own breath and drop into the body to really feel the message and truly listen to the story it has to tell, we create the space for our own healing and transformation. Deep, yogic breathing is the most effective way to access this story. Yogic breathing renews and restores every cell of our being and cleanses and detoxifies the nervous system. As you practice slow, steady, smooth, deep and even breathing, notice if your mind is becoming quieter and more placid and content. When we consciously and intentionally move toward more complete exhalations and deeper, fuller inhalations, we create more expansive space in the physical body which contributes to the emotional and psychological experience of relaxation and ease.

Conscious breathing is one of the most readily accessible ways to navigate the emotional waves of grief

As I write these paragraphs about yogic breathing, my family is grieving the loss of my son's dog, Kirby. Kirby was my son's first dog, and the first sentient being that my son and daughter-in-law cared for together. They adopted him and gave him a home for 11 years. Kirby was a faithful friend, companion, and protector of all of us who are part of his "pack," and he adapted kindly, patiently, and gently to the presence of the little children who have been born into his family.

As I practiced yoga this morning, my mind was flooded with thoughts and memories of this dog whom I love. Waves of emotions came with those memories. In an effort to ride the waves, I focused more intently on my breath, especially in the quieter moments of my yoga practice. I created a pattern of breathing that was slightly more complicated in order to hold my attention on the breath, inhaling to a count of four, gently pausing the breath for two counts, and exhaling to a count of six. The stories and memories of Kirby are important; I was not avoiding them or denying them. Rather, I was using a breathing technique to gently and compassionately honor and release the heavy energy of the emotions associated with my memories and my grief.

Grounding and centering technique: guided conscious relaxation in a restorative posture

In periods of transition from one state of being to another, grounding and centering is a way to anchor ourselves in the experience of the present moment, letting go of the burdens of the past and anxiety about the future.

For this practice of conscious relaxation, please clothe yourself so that you can be comfortably warm, or have a blanket handy to cover yourself once you have settled in. The body cools down as it relaxes, and if you are too cold you will be uncomfortable and distracted. If it is useful to you, you may wish to record the sound of your own voice guiding you through this grounding and centering technique. Feel free to adapt it and make it your own. Find language that feels authentic for you.

Begin by finding a supported, balanced posture that feels good and comfortable. I suggest reclining on the ground, close to the earth, but you might recline or sit on a piece of furniture. Teacher and choreographer, Abraham Remy Charlip, said, "When in doubt, get horizontal." Use *savasana*, the corpse pose, at the beginning, in the middle, or at the end of a yoga practice, or as a practice in and of itself. It is a practice of *isvara pranidhana*, or surrender. Give over to gravity and the support of the earth.

When we are in utero, completely sheltered and safe in our mother's womb, we are curled up with every joint in flexion. When we bring the joints into flexion by supporting the knees on a bolster or blanket roll and supporting the head on a folded blanket or small pillow, we mimic this primordial posture of safety and security. The spine is aligned and the support under the knees releases tension in the low back. The support under the head allows the chin to be slightly tucked so that the forehead is higher than the chin. This head position cues the nervous system to relax and drop toward a parasympathetic state.

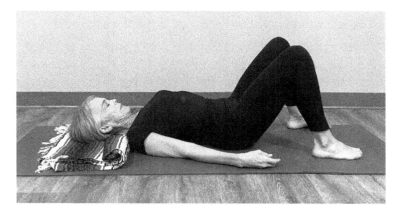

Once you have reclined, adjust each limb of the body. Lift one leg, hug the knee toward your chest, rock the knee side to side, wiggle your toes and make circles with the foot and ankle in both directions. Then stretch the foot far away from your heart and allow the leg to rest on the floor. Make similar adjustments with your other leg until you feel both legs resting in equanimity on the earth.

Now adjust your shoulders and arms. Hug yourself. As you do so, say words of loving kindness toward yourself.

Let the words be authentic to you. Reach your own finger tips toward your shoulder blades on the back of your body and broaden the space behind your heart by adjusting your shoulders on the steady, reliable ground. Unwrap one arm from your chest and reach it away from you. Wiggle the fingers and make circles with the hand and wrist. Then allow the bones of the arms to rest in a neutral position. Rest the arm on the earth or on your body, so the thumb turns toward your heart and the pinkie finger rest on the earth or on your body. Adjust the other arm in a similar fashion. Rock the head side to side, bringing one ear toward the earth and then the other. Once you have adjusted your limbs and head, ask yourself, "Is there anything further I can do to make myself five-to-ten percent more comfortable?" and adjust accordingly. Seek to release any muscular contraction that would attempt to hold your posture in any particular way.

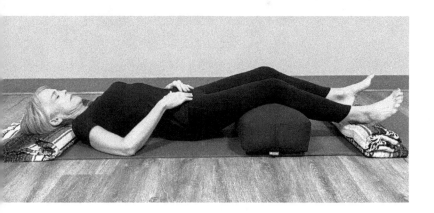

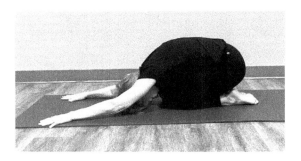

In this space of comfort, allow your body to rest motionless, not holding still, but being still. If you become uncomfortable, feel free to move into child's pose or crocodile pose (lying prostrate on the body of the earth) or a side-lying *savasana*. If you need to move, move mindfully, and to the best of your ability, maintain an easy, steady breathing pattern. Allow space for your own emotion.

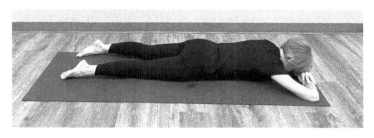

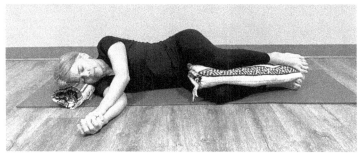

Feel your body resting heavily and comfortably on the body of the earth. Feel the parts of the body that are heavy and dense, related to the energy of the earth. Allow your body weight to release under the pull of gravity. Imagine the earth rising to support you, or cradle you, as you continue to release, finding more comfort and stability. You are resting on the ground, the reliable, stable body of the earth.

Feel the parts of the body that are spacious and light, related to the energy of air and wind. Notice the prevailing wind of the body, the rhythm of your breath. Bring conscious awareness to the sensations of your breath. Notice how long it takes you to inhale, notice if there is a natural pause after you inhale. Notice how long it takes you to exhale, and notice if there is a natural space of emptiness after you exhale. Just follow the breath, without trying to fix it or force it in any specific way.

Use a grounding breath to release more fully.

- ✽ Inhale through the nose, and exhale through an open mouth using a sighing sound/ Release the weight of the physical body.
- ✽ Inhale through the nose, and exhale through an open mouth using a sighing sound/ Release the weight of the mind.
- ✽ Inhale through the nose, and exhale through an open mouth using a sighing sound/ Release the weight of the world.

❋ To better release the weight of the mind, bring awareness to the past. Take note of whatever things are standing out in your memory now. Review the things that you've heard or said, done or accomplished. Recall the feelings you've had.

If you are recording this narrative, allow a pause here, leaving time for and inventory of your thoughts.

❋ Now ask the mind to put all of that on hold behind you, trusting that, if you need those memories, they will be there for you.

❋ Bring into your mind the events of the future, events awaiting you later today or this week or this month. Notice any thoughts or feelings that you have about the future.

If you are recording this narrative, allow a pause here, leaving time for and inventory of your thoughts.

❋ Now ask the mind to put all of that on hold in front of you, trusting that, when we arrive in the future, all will be well.

❋ Now you are free to step more fully into this present moment and be present in this practice. If it resonates as truthful or meaningful for you, you might silently repeat this *mantra* to yourself: "Inhaling I come home. Exhaling I arrive." If the mind wanders off, simply bring it back to the breath and the *mantra*.

Inhaling I come home. Exhaling I arrive.

You can use this phrase as a *mantra* at any time during the day. If you notice that feelings of agitation or fear or irritation or anger are present, use your breath or a *mantra* as a tool to prevent the feelings from taking control of you.

Allow the heart and throat to rest openly, and bring one hand to rest on your heart and the other to rest on your belly. As you feel the breath drop into the body and the body drop into the breath, can you begin to gently manipulate the breath so that it passes through the nose, the throat, the chest, and then changes the shape of the belly as you inhale? As you exhale, lightly contract the muscles of the pelvic floor and lift the pelvic floor toward the navel and the navel toward the spine. By moderately drawing the belly toward the spine on the exhalation, you create the natural opportunity for the body to rebound on the inhalation and receive the breath through the nose, throat, chest, and then allowing the shape-change in the belly. Notice the corresponding parts of the back body also expanding as you inhale. Feel the back of the neck lengthen and relax, the back of the heart broaden and the low back release on the support of the earth as your body receives breath to restore and renew every cell. Work mindfully with the exhalation, allowing the belly to drop toward the spine. A deeper, fuller inhalation may naturally follow.

If you notice that your belly contracts on the inhalation, you may have a habit of reverse breathing. Reverse breathing is a habit that may be borne from chronic fear or stress. If you suspect that you are reverse breathing, bring both hands to your low belly and as you exhale tenderly push down with your hands to coax the breath out. Working with our breath is working with our life – one breath in and one breath out. We work in a spirit of gentleness and compassion to heal every cell and every part of our being.

> ❄ *Inhale the serenity to accept the things you cannot change.*
> ❄ *Exhale fear, doubt, worry, and anxiety.*
> ❄ *Inhale the courage to change the things you can.*
> ❄ *Exhale anger, frustration, impatience, despair.*
> ❄ *Inhale the wisdom to know the difference.*
> ❄ *Exhale self-doubt.*
> ❄ *Repeat.*

You may conclude your practice here or continue with the practice of progressive relaxation. When you are completely finished resting in *savasana*, please curl up on one side in the fetal position and pause for several cycles of breath before gently moving to a comfortable seated position.

Body scan and progressive relaxation

The following is one method of the practice of progressive relaxation. There are many methods for this practice, but I prefer methods in which the body remains motionless, and the consciousness is rotated without introducing movement into the physical body. Movement, no matter how small, creates muscular contraction. This, in my experience, is counter-productive in relaxation practices. But your experience may be different than mine, so feel free to adapt it and make it your own.

Resting in a comfortable reclining position that feels balanced, supported, and spacious, allow yourself to breathe deeply. Draw the breath into the lowest lobes of the lungs as you inhale, and exhale fully and completely. Bring your awareness to the point between the eyebrows, in the mid-brain, behind the center of the forehead and above the soft palate of the mouth. Visualize light. Notice the color and intensity of the light. As you inhale you might see the light expand and as you exhale, you might see the light soften.

From the point between the eyebrows, direct the light of your awareness down into your feet. Visualize your feet at the point between the eyebrows. Visualize the bones, joints, muscles, tendons, ligaments, and skin of your feet. Inhale and, in your imagination, illuminate your feet, and as you exhale, invite a greater sense of ease and relaxation into your feet.

Now bring your awareness back to the point between the eyebrows, and from that energetic center, direct the light of your awareness into your ankles and calves. Visualize the bones, joints, muscles, tendons, ligaments, and skin of your ankles and calves. Inhale deeply and, in your imagination, illuminate your ankles and calves, and as you exhale, invite a greater sense of ease and relaxation into your ankles and calves.

From the point between the eyebrows, direct the light of your awareness into your thighs and hips. Visualize the bones, joints, muscles, tendons, ligaments, and skin of your thighs and hips. Inhale deeply and, in your imagination, illuminate your thighs and hips. With your exhalation, invite release and relaxation into your thighs and hips.

From the point between the eyebrows, direct the light of your awareness into your entire spine. Visualize your entire spine, from the tip of the coccyx, through the five fused vertebrae of your sacral spine, through the five articulating vertebrae of your lumber spine, your low back, through the 12 articulating vertebrae of your thoracic spine, the part of your spine that's behind your heart and connected to your ribs, through the seven vertebrae of your cervical spine, your neck, including the atlas supporting the base of your skull. Illuminate your entire spine, every bone, disc, and all the connective tissue. See your spine, radiant with light. As you inhale, visualize your entire spine lengthening. As you exhale, invite the energy of relaxation into your entire spine and feel the spine soften and release.

From the point between the eyebrows, direct the light of your awareness into the root of your spine and your pelvis.

Visualize your pelvis. See the bones, joints, muscles, tendons, ligaments, and skin. Visualize the internal organs, organs of reproduction and elimination. Feel the heavy bones of the pelvis and connect with a sense of heaviness, or earthiness. Feel the fluidity of your breath and connect with a sense of ease, flow, and pleasure. Inhale and, in your imagination, see the root of your spine and your pelvis, illuminated, bathed in light. As you exhale, invite the energy of relaxation to flood your pelvis.

From the point between the eyebrows, direct the light of your awareness into your whole abdomen and the corresponding parts of the back body. See the internal organs, the digestive system, the liver, the spleen, the pancreas and the gallbladder. See the kidneys and adrenals in the deepest part of the abdomen. See the muscles and skin of the belly. Inhale into the intelligent and powerful center of your belly, and in your mind's eye, see it fully illuminated. Then, as you exhale, invite the belly to completely release and relax.

From the point between the eyebrows, direct the light of your awareness into the energetic center of your heart. Illuminate the center of the chest, and allow that light to flood the entire chest, the bones, muscles and tissue of the area around the sternum and ribs. Illuminate the vital organs, the muscle of the heart, all five lobes of the of the lungs, and the circulatory system. Allow the light to spill and flood the shoulders and upper back, the arms, from the head of each humerus down to the tip of every finger. Bathe your heart in light. Notice if there is any heaviness resting on the energetic center of the heart. Notice if there is any weight or darkness resting on the light of the heart. Be aware of any feelings of sadness, fear, or disappointment.

> ❀ *Breath one, inhale*: As you breathe in through your nostrils, use your breath to lift any sadness, heaviness, and darkness off of the heart. In your mind's eye, see the heaviness lift up off of the heart like a cloud.
>
> ❀ *Breath one, exhale*: Now as you exhale, disperse that heaviness out into the universe through the nostrils. Imagine that you can see it like soot or smoke.
>
> ❀ *Breath two, inhale*: The next time you inhale, see light from the heavens and draw the light into your heart. Inhale healing love into your heart.
>
> ❀ *Breath two, exhale*: Now as you exhale, anchor the love in your heart. In your mind, see healing love flood your heart with light.
>
> ❀ *Repeat.*
>
> ❀ Repeat this two breath cycle numerous times until you feel light and spaciousness flooding your heart. At a certain point, you might feel that you are no longer "visualizing" or "doing" the practice; rather, you've entered it.
>
> ❀ *If you are recording this narrative, allow a pause here, leaving time for the repetition of this four-part, two-breath practice for the energetic center of the heart.*

Now direct the light of your awareness into the energetic center of your throat. From the point between the eyebrows, illuminate your throat with healing light. Visualize your throat, inner and outer, the bone of the jaw, the mouth, the lips, the tongue, the teeth, the hard and soft palette of the mouth, the inner ear and outer ears, and the internal organs, the thyroid and parathyroid. Feel the bone of the jaw resting heavily in the flesh of the face. Feel the lips resting softly, maybe slightly parted. Inhale light into the entire energetic region of the throat. As you breathe in through the nostrils, imagine drawing breath in through your ears as well. Inhale, creating the image of radiant light in the energetic center of the throat, and, as you exhale, invite a sense of relaxation to abide there.

From the point between the eyebrows, direct the light of your awareness into your face, your skull and your brain. In your mind's eye, see your radiant, illuminated face and bathe the skull and brain in light. See your face resting, soft, at ease, without tension. Inhale healing light into your face, skull, and brain, and, as you exhale, invite the light to abide there.

Finally, visualize your whole body resting on the body of the earth. From the point between your eyebrows, see your whole body. Illuminate your whole body with radiant, healing light. Bathe yourself in light. Inhale into your whole body, and as you exhale, invite your entire body to find more release, more serenity, more relaxation.

You may rest in the benefits of this simple practice of progressive relaxation as long as you wish. When you are completely finished resting in savasana, please curl up on one side in the fetal position and pause for several cycles of breath before gently moving to a comfortable seated position to either continue your practice or continue your day.

Body scan with the word "GRIEF"

Set up: For this body scan practice, I recommend using a supported reclining pose. You might choose to extend the legs with a bolster behind the knees, or you might prefer *supta bandha konasana*. If you have a yoga block and a bolster, you can use the props to elevate your head and heart so the chest opens and the back of the heart is supported. Please be sure that your lower back is completely comfortable at all times. The sacrum should rest close to the bolster to prevent compression in the lowest parts of the spine. You might roll up a blanket or towel to adjust the angle of your body on the bolster. Use pillows, blankets, cushions, and props to create spacious support for your body and mind. Once you have

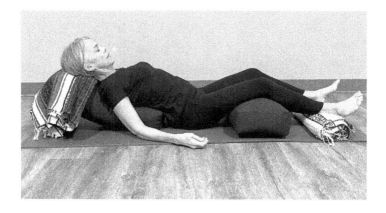

your props and your body situated, allow yourself several cycles of deep, diaphragmatic breathing to settle in.

Body scan: We tend to transfer or carry the pain from our loss in specific parts of our body. When you hear the word "GRIEF," notice the sensations in your physical body.

Is there one part of the body that particularly vibrates, resonates, closes, contracts, or collapses when you hear or say the word "GRIEF?" Direct your full awareness to that place. You might put one hand immediately on that part of the body. Keeping your hand there, or imagining the weight of your hand there, take slow, deep breaths, and visualize light, breathing into the space beneath your hand. As you breathe into the space under your hand, notice if the energy of the space changes. Is there a color that arises in your internal gaze? Do you hear any internal sound as you breathe into the space? Flood the area with breath and healing light and energy. Allow some time here.

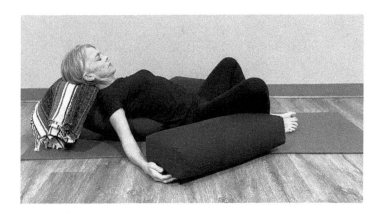

Is there another space in your body quietly asking for your attention? Either direct your awareness or place your other hand there. Continue to breathe for several minutes into the space beneath your hands. Circulate breath and light and healing energy into these spaces and into every cell of your body.

After several minutes in this pose, deepen the breath. When you feel as though the practice is complete, on a full exhalation, slowly roll your body to one side. Rest in the fetal position here for several breaths before gently making your way to a seated position.

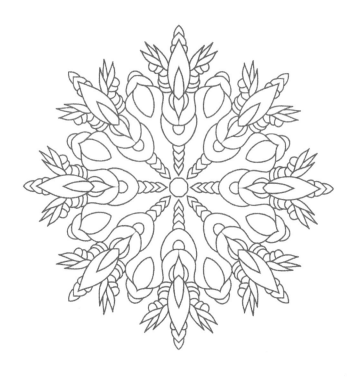

Pelvic tilts and dynamic bridge pose – linking breath and movement

Grief can feel like a heavy burden. It's not unusual for our posture to change when our hearts are heavy with sadness and grief. We might let our head hang, hunch down, and look down toward the ground. Our shoulders might slump and roll inward, the upper spine might round, and the chest might begin to collapse. This is the body's posture in protection mode; it as though we are trying to shield our hearts from further pain and suffering.

There are times when it is indeed appropriate to shield our hearts and retreat into our shell, but if a slumping posture becomes habitual and chronic, it can affect the lungs and heart, leading to breathing difficulties and fatigue. Digestive problems can even occur, as well as neurological problems if the nerves in the spine are compressed.

This dynamic bridge sequence is designed as a soothing method of opening the entire front line of the body, including the lungs and the energetic center of the heart. Because all of the chambers of the lungs expand in this pose and sequence, it is a gentle way to introduce movement to the body if you are feeling fatigue and lethargy. It is also a pacifying way to comfort yourself if you are feeling symptoms of anxiety, as the moderate elevation of the heart above the head will be quieting to the brain.

Bridge pose both strengthens the muscles of the back body and releases tension in the muscles of the back.

Practicing this posture gives us the physical experience of standing in power and authority on our own two feet, with an open heart and supple neck. This may sound like a tall order when our heart is broken, but the gentle practice of these postures can truly lighten our emotional load.

Dynamic variations are included here, moving the arms and head to relieve stress and tension in the neck and shoulders. Mindful attention to the "choreography" of this sequence will require focus of the mind and strengthen the breath-brain connection. The sequence begins gently. Remember, less is more. If you experience pain anywhere, please back off and do less, yet continue on for yourself.

Bridge sequence

Lie on your back. Bend your knees and stand the soles of your feet on the ground, placing them in a position that allows you to access the strength and power of your legs. Feel your feet and back body on the ground, connecting to the stable, reliable energy of the earth. Feel the sole of each foot connect with the earth and balance the weight in each foot over the arch. Lift all ten toes, wiggle them and rest them back on the earth with the big toes facing straight forward. Feel the ball mount of each toe rooted and connected. Feel the center of each heel anchored, and know that you are grounded in your own personal authority.

As you connect through the soles of the feet, connect with the strength of all sides of each thigh and internally rotate each femur head (thigh bone) in your hip sockets so you feel your inner thighs spin down to the earth. You might place a small yoga block between your thighs to fortify the sensation of the inner rotation of the femurs. If you use a block, feel the entire surface of the inner thigh spiraling evenly into the block. As the femurs internally rotate, you might feel the low belly lightly engage. This intentional placement of the bones engages the bandhas.

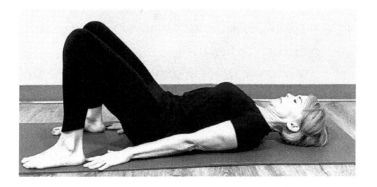

Place your hands on the ground, palms down, outside your hips. Spread the fingers and actively press your hands into the ground. Let your hands be part of your experience of becoming grounded. Do you feel the muscles of the arms engage? Your hands and arms are related to the energetic center of your heart. These are the hands you use to express kindness through acts of service, compassion and affection. As you exhale, root your hands into the earth. As you inhale, invite the energy of loving kindness up through your arms into the center of your heart.

Now, as you exhale, imprint your waistband into the earth. You might feel the abdominal wall lengthen, hollow, and engage. This is your core, your center of power and emotional intelligence. Inhale and soften the abdomen, allowing the lower back to return to its natural curve. Repeat this action, pressing the waistband into the ground as you exhale and releasing the tilt of the pelvis as you inhale, linking the breath and movement. Do this several times, allowing this simple action to connect you with the steady rhythm of your breath. Notice that you have power to restrain and control the breath, and also to allow it to flow freely.

When you are ready, as you exhale, lengthen the back body on the earth and press into all corners of the feet to lift the pelvis off the floor, sliding it onto your strong, sturdy legs for bridge pose. Inhale in bridge pose, releasing the tuck of the pelvis and feeling the weight of your pelvis anchored on your legs. As the entire abdominal wall lengthens, shine the light of your power and truth. As you exhale, deepen the pelvic tilt and lower the spine to the earth. Imagine releasing the spine vertebra by vertebra, from the voice box down to the tailbone. Reconnect with the steady energy of the earth, inhaling here and softening the abdomen. Repeat this cycle several times. Then rest for a few full cycles of breath and receive the energy of the pose.

Next, leaving the back body resting on the ground, exhale and imprint the spine on the earth and as you inhale, allow the breath to lift the right arm over head, turning the face to the left, away from the arm. The belly will soften as you reach the arm overhead, but allow the frontal ribs to rest in the body. Let your exhalation bring your face back to center, your arm back to your side, and press your back body into the ground. Inhale in this neutral position, softening the front body, and then exhale, imprint your spine on the earth and allow your next inhalation to lift your left arm over head turning your face to the right, away from your uplifted arm. Repeat this two times more on each side.

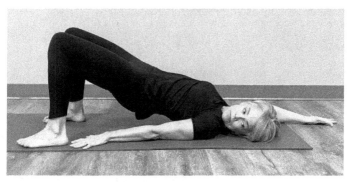

Finally, combine steps one and two of this "dance," so that as you exhale, you imprint your back body on the earth. Your inhalation will simultaneously lift your pelvis off the ground and onto your strong legs as your right arm lifts over head and your face turns to the left. Your exhalation will bring everything back to the starting position. Then inhale and soften the front body, filling the nose, throat, chest, and belly with breath. Exhale, imprint your spine on the ground and allow your inhalation to lift your left arm over head as your spine lengthens and your pelvis lifts. Your face will turn to the right, away from the arm. Then your exhalation will bring your whole body back to resolution in the position where you began. Repeat this action four or five more times on each side for a total of five or six rounds. Rest for two full cycles of breath before rolling to one side, pressing your way to a comfortable seat, and then coming to standing. Please note that as you move from reclined to seated and then standing, your blood pressure needs time to adjust to the different positions of your head in relationship to your heart. Please breathe deeply as you make this transition.

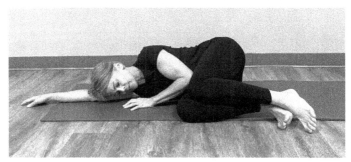

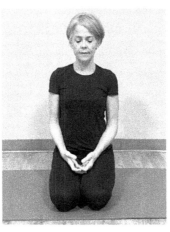

Standing postures to turn down the stress response

Take your time to really feel your own alignment and position in every one of the following standing poses. Doing this will help to train your mind to be attentive and relaxed and will develop your proprioception. Scientific research has shown that increasing proprioceptive input with balance and movement practices like yoga actually reduces sympathetic nervous system activation, effectively turning down the stress response and reducing anxiety.

Tadasana: mountain pose, option of a wall at your back

Practicing a tall, strong *tadasana* every day can be a great remedy to counteract the effects of grief on your posture. I especially enjoy practicing the pose with a wall at my back. The practice of *tadasana*, or mountain pose, is literally the practice of standing in power on our own two feet with steadiness, comfort, courage, and grace. This is beneficial to all of the *chakras* and every aspect of our being – physical, emotional, energetic, and spiritual.

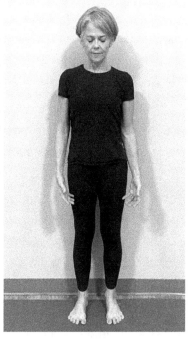

Feel both of your feet standing firmly on the earth. Stand with your toes headed in the same direction your knees are facing. This helps to stabilize the knees. Imagine that the sturdy soles of the feet contain a tripod which includes the center of each heel, the ball mount of each big toe and the ball mount of each baby toe. Press the tripods of your feet actively into the ground and feel for the sensation of the arches of the feet lifting and activating. Move the inner ankles back, outer ankles in, outer shins in. This attention without tension in the feet and lower extremities helps to activate and balance the root *chakra*.

To stand with authority, we create the intention to internally rotate the big, strong bones of the thighs in the hip sockets. This moves energy to the mid-line of the body and activates our center. You might again place a small yoga block between your thighs to fortify the sensation of the internal rotation of the femurs. With the thigh bones rotated inward, we might then imagine moving the heads of the thigh bones back in their sockets so the pelvic basin can rest solidly on the strong, sturdy bones of the legs. This activates *mula bandha*.

Now find buoyancy and good space in the joints and note the watery quality of the pelvis, keeping it neutral. This is nourishing for the second *chakra*.

The natural curves of the human spine provide a beautiful image for understanding strength and stability in a new way. Our spine is strongest and most stable when we stand in our natural curves. Without working too hard to change anything about the natural flow of the curves in our spine, we stand in our strength and power. With the tailbone in a neutral position, the pubic bone dropping toward the earth, and the sternum lifting toward heaven, the easy, gentle curves of the neck and low back flow in unaltered grace.

Externally rotate the bones of the upper arm and take them slightly back to expand the chest into the pits of the arms. Draw the shoulder blades toward the spine and feel them soften down the back, toward the waist. Create space for something new in the energetic region of the heart.

If you are practicing this pose with the wall at your back, feel the sensation of something solid and stable behind you; the wall literally has your back. Soften all the muscles of your face, and close you eyes if you are comfortable. Breathe deeply.

❀ *Who or what in this world has your back to support you today?*

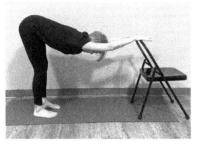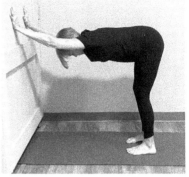

Adho mukha svanasana/Downward facing dog pose using a wall or the back of a chair

Place your hands on the wall or on the back of the chair approximately the same width as your shoulders. Slowly walk your feet back away from the wall or chair, and slide your hands down if you are using the wall. Bring your body into the shape of a sideways letter "L." The legs need not be absolutely straight. Instead, search for a sensation of opening in the entire back line of the body. Create height and length in the spine and notice the opening in the front line of the torso as well.

A certain amount of mindful fidgeting here may help to release muscular tension, and when you are ready, settle into a stable, still pose and breathe deeply. Notice any inclination to try to perfect or change the posture. Notice the mind, notice the breath, and stay with what is happening in the present moment. When you are ready to come out of the pose, deepen your breath, slowly walk your feet towards the wall or the chair, and inhale as you stand upright.

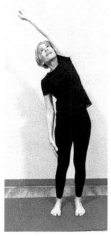 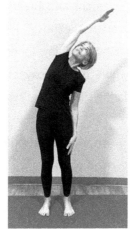 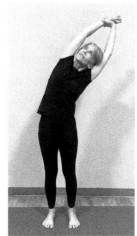

Tadasana with lateral spinal stretch

Strength, power, suppleness, and ease are expressed as we extend one or both arms up, and flex the spine to the right. If both arms are overhead, you might clasp the hands and gently pull your left wrist with your right hand. Feel the opening in the side of the rib cage, and breathe deeply into all the chambers of the lungs for several breaths.

Is grief stored in the lungs? It can definitely impair our breathing. Expand your exhalations and inhalations to free this region of your body from tension. Pause in tadasana before switching sides. When you take the posture on the left side, notice the subtle differences between the two sides of the body.

Breath of Joy is a movement and breath sequence, with a three-part inhale through the nose, and a long exhale through the mouth, making a sighing sound. This practice is fun! It awakens your whole system, oxygenating the blood, and temporarily stimulating the nervous system.

Breath of Joy can be modified and practiced while seated on a chair. It may not be appropriate for everyone, even in a modified version. If you have high blood pressure, or if you suffer from any kind of head or eye injury, migraines, or glaucoma, you might modify it or skip it. If you start to feel light-headed, instead of light-hearted, stop for a minute and just breathe normally. You may take the sequence in half-time, as your breath allows.

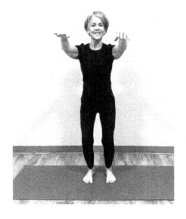
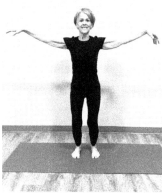

Begin by standing away from the wall with your feet a little wider than hip width apart. Feel your feet on the ground, and let your knees be buoyant. For the three-part inhale through the nose:

1) Take a short inhale as you lift your arms forward in front of your body.

2) Take another short inhale as you lift your arms out to the sides of the body.

3) Take a third, slightly longer inhale as you raise your arms up overhead.

4) Then take a long exhale through the mouth, making a clearly audible sighing sound, and lean your torso out over your legs, releasing your arms and head toward the earth. Do not be shy creating the sound.

Repeat this sequence up to nine times. Then take a long exhale....

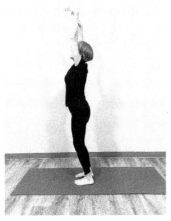
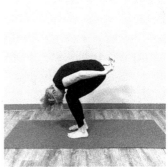

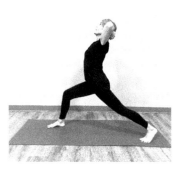 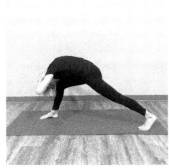

Banner and shield sequence

If this sequence is not accessible standing, it may be practiced while seated on a chair, omitting the warrior lunge. If you choose to practice it standing and balance feels precarious, create a broader base of support left to right, so each foot is in its own lane on the mat, and feet are not arranged as on a balance beam. For added stability, you may stand with your back heel against the wall.

From *tadasana*, step the right foot forward to come into a high crescent lunge. If you are practicing this sequence on a chair, take a tall seat at the edge of the chair. This is a two-breath, four-part sequence, to be repeated several times.

✻ *Breath one, inhale:* Interlace the fingers at the back of the skull. Take a deep breath in through the nose and as you do lift the back of your skull into the support of your hands. Open the front line of your body – your throat, chest and belly – and draw into your being whatever you are bringing into your life today.

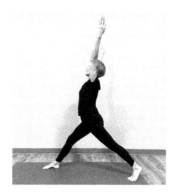 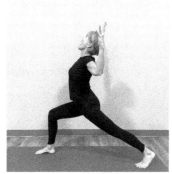

❋ *Breath one, exhale*: As you exhale, draw your belly button to your spine and push the breath out completely through your mouth. Round your back body, lower your chin toward your chest, and bow your head toward your bent front knee. With the back body rounded, go into your shell. This is tortoise energy. Shield yourself from behaviors and patterns that no longer serve you. Allow them to be behind you. Consciously move out the energy of whatever you are putting to rest, whatever no longer serves you. Modify or adapt the flexion of your spine as it is appropriate for you.

❋ *Breath two, inhale*: Inhale through the nostrils, and as you breathe in rise up, straighten the front leg, reach your arms toward heaven in the shape of a wide "V." Imagine that you are holding a banner of victory! Open your throat and chest and draw the breath in fully.

✼ *Breath two, exhale*: Exhale, bend the front knee and both elbows making a "W" shape with the arms. Open your chest and roar a mighty lion's breath. With the mouth wide open, stick your tongue out of your mouth and eyes out of your head and create a roaring sound that rises all the way from your pelvic floor. This clears every *chakra* from the root to the throat.

Repeat this sequence for six to ten rounds on the right side. You may notice shifting sensations – the feeling of being on or off balance – and extraneous thoughts may take you away from your movements. Simplify the movements as needed, and emphasize the practice of the breath. This will improve mental focus in general, both on and off the yoga mat. After practicing on the right side, stand in *tadasana* or sit tall for several cycles of breath before repeating on the left side. Then stand in *tadasana* or sit tall and breathe.

"Courage is the most important of all the
virtues, because without courage you
can't practice any other virtue consistently.
You can practice any virtue erratically,
but nothing consistently without courage."
~ Maya Angelou

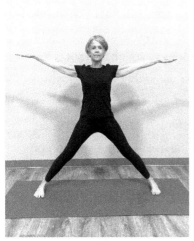 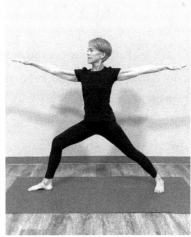

Warrior II

Step the feet wide on the mat, about three or four feet apart. Begin with the feet parallel or slightly pigeon-toed. Life doesn't consistently bestow the blessed opportunity to stand on solid ground, so in this moment notice how wonderful it feels as you stand on the steady earth and on your own two feet. Acknowledge the strength and power of your legs and stand in your authority with an open heart. Even with the feet wide, stand firmly on both feet, so that the ankles and weight-bearing joints of the legs are not collapsed or uncomfortable.

Come into Warrior II on the right side, turning your right toes toward the short end of your mat. Angle your left heel out a few degrees, so your left big toe is directed slightly toward your right foot. See that your right heel is approximately on line with the back arch of your left foot. Bend your right knee in the direction of the center of your right foot, not past the joint of the ankle to help prevent the collapse of your left leg. In every standing yoga pose, your back leg is the power of the posture and your back foot is the anchor of the pose, so keep your whole back foot pressing firmly into the ground and your back leg straight and strong as a steel rod. Keep the spine tall and reach your arms out wide, wrists online with the shoulders. Be aware of the position of your body in space. Is your head really aligned over the root of your spine? Turn the palms toward the ground, and focus your gaze out over your right finger tips. Your vision might slightly blur as you gaze intently. This gazing practice reminds us that we cannot always clearly see what is before us. It is at least partially a mystery. But we can fearlessly stand, fully grounded in the present moment, with all sides of the heart open. The front side of the heart center is concerned with what is before us. The left and right sides of the heart center are concerned with our relationships with others. The back side of the energetic center of the heart is concerned with the past. Are there experiences in the past that need to be forgiven? Are there people that we need to forgive, for the sake of our own wellbeing and peace of mind? Do we need to forgive ourselves?

Standing face to face with mystery, including the mystery of suffering, looking into the unknown, and maintaining an open heart is my personal definition of the spiritual warrior. As we face grief squarely, we stay focused and committed to our resolve to not allow grief to overtake us.

"I am grateful to be courageous, loving, vulnerable, strong." Our resolve is not a cure all, but it can help us to explore grief, to probe it and know it personally.

Now create the posture on the left side. Each new side is a brand new event. Create the posture with attention to your alignment and be respectful of the subtle differences in the right and left sides of your body.

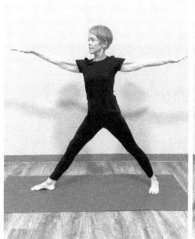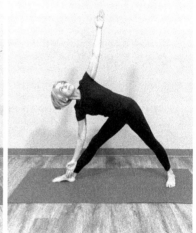

Trikonasana, Triangle pose

After practicing Warrior II on the right and the left side, return to your wide-legged stance. Turn your right toes to the short end of the mat once more, aligning your right heel with the back arch of your left foot. Keep the right leg straight but the knee unlocked. Keep the heart open, keep all sides of the spine long, and tip your torso toward the right leg for triangle pose.

Triangle pose provides an ideal combination of opening, elongating, stretching, and challenging the body. The deep stretch through the body can help to release tension and promote relaxation without dullness.

Bring mindful awareness to your alignment and position in space. Again, this helps to train the mind and develop and improve proprioception, which reduces sympathetic nervous system activation, turning down the stress response and reducing anxiety.

Stay in *trikonasana* for several breaths. Triangle is an effective and rejuvenating yoga posture to create equilibrium between the mind and body. It balances the root *chakra*, second (sacral) *chakra*, and heart *chakra*. Inhale to come out of the pose, and then bring the feet parallel before setting up for triangle pose on the left side.

Step both feet together in *tadasana* at the top of the mat or with a wall at your back. Stand and receive for several cycles of breath. Fully integrate into every breath and every cell of your being your intention and resolve to create space for and receive what is most beneficial for your wholeness, wellness, health, and vitality.

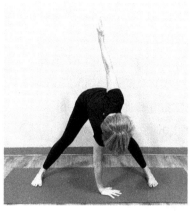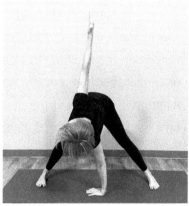

Prasarita Padottanasana (wide stance forward fold) and twisting _trikonasana_

This dynamic sequence includes an ancient variation of revolved triangle pose, which resembles a windmill. Use the wind of your breath to powerfully direct this sequence. The poses can be modified by using the back or seat of a chair for support instead of bending toward the ground.

As you inhale, come to stand in a wide legged position with your feet about three or four feet apart. Begin with the feet parallel or slightly pigeon-toed. Again, stand on the tripods of each foot, so that the ankles and weight-bearing joints of the legs are not collapsed or uncomfortable.

Focus your awareness at the navel center through this sequence. Exhale, and imagine energy moving down from your navel, through your legs, into the soles of your feet. Bring the hands to the hips as you inhale, and exhale to fold forward placing your hands on the earth, or use blocks or a chair to bring the earth to you.

Inhaling, bring your left hand to the middle of your space, and exhale to spin your left rib cage toward your right inner thigh. Allow the right hand to rest at the sacrum or extend the right arm toward the sky. Inhale to find more length and space, and then exhale and switch sides. Inhale here, and switch again. Continue moving with your breath. Move as quickly or as slowly as your breath and your body inspire you to move. Slower movement may increase focus and be more calming. Faster movement might be more energizing and invigorating. Listen to *your* body as you move through each pose. Connect with the natural flow and rhythm of your breath. On every exhalation, lift the pelvic floor to the navel and draw the navel toward the spine to support and fortify your low back. Notice the stability you create for yourself through the conscious use of your breath and focused awareness in the center of your body. As you inhale, expand the heart in six directions – up, down, left, right, front, and back. Twist right and then left six or seven times.

If you are practicing this windmill sequence with a group, you might spontaneously synchronize your movements with the other people in the room. Notice how breathing and moving together with a group increases your sense of connection with others.

After six or seven complete rounds, linking breath and movement, rest in the center. When you are ready to come out of the forward fold, breathe in deeply as you rise. Inhaling on the way up from a forward fold helps to regulate blood pressure and prevent dizziness, so you might rise up only part way on an inhalation, pause and exhale, and then rise up the rest of the way as you inhale again. Exhale here. If your inner legs need a rest from this wide stance, step the feet together.

The image of a windmill can serve as one metaphor for the grieving process. The mysterious force of the wind powers a windmill, just as the mysterious force of grief can create a churning in the depths of our being. As a windmill utilizes the unpredictable and sometimes destructive force of the wind into constructive energy, the techniques of our yoga practice – conscious breathing, postures, meditation, and reflection – can transform our experiences of the forces of the unknown, of death and rebirth, into deeper understanding of our eternal self.

Wide stance downward facing dog with head supported
Return to a wide stance when you feel ready. Have props ready: a bolster, a block, a blanket, pillow, or chair. Exhale to fold forward, and walk your hands forward so that your spine is in the shape of downward facing dog. Create a wide-stance downward facing dog, with your heels on the ground. If possible, allow your forehead to rest on the earth or on a prop.

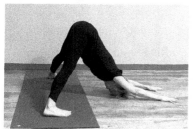 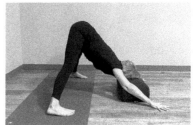

We don't just get over grief. Instead, we change our relationship to it.

Subordinating the head to the heart in an inverted pose, we have the opportunity to shift our perspective. We are here, rooted in the present moment, standing firm on our own two legs. We look respectfully back at all that is behind us, and that which is in front of us is a mystery. Supported and strong, feel the strength of your legs and core facilitating the opening around your heart and the lengthening on all sides of your spine. Practice trust.

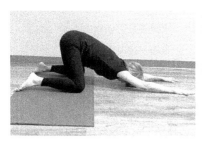 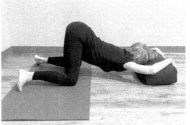

Anahata balasana **to** *bhujangasana,* **puppy/cobra pose**

From this wide stance, downward facing dog, lower your knees to the earth. Start with your hips over knees, arms extended. Draw the sit-bones halfway back towards your calves as you resist with the palms, pressing into the floor to lengthen the spine and back muscles.

Breathe into the back of your heart. Imagine someone's hand on your back, lifting your heart through the front of your chest. Hold for several full cycles of breath. Maintain the length on all sides of your spine as you inhale and slowly slide forward into cobra pose. Allow all sides of your neck to be long. Exhale and slide back to puppy pose. Soften the space around your heart even more. Repeat this sequence for six or more cycles of breath. Then rest in child's pose or some other comfortable position and receive.

The heavy emotional energy of grief can create pain and tension around the entire energetic center of the heart and throat. These simple, accessible seated postures and movements serve to release that tension.

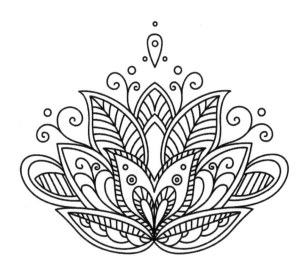

"One of the most beautiful gifts in the world is the gift of encouragement. When someone encourages you, that person helps you over a threshold you might otherwise never have crossed on your own."
~John O'Donohue

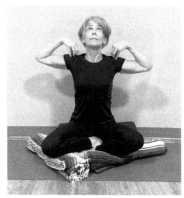

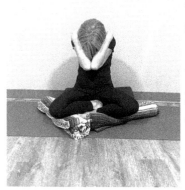

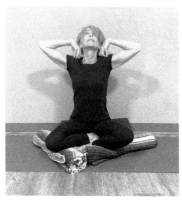

"Butterfly wings" pose

Come to sit in a comfortable position on the floor, on a block or blanket, or sit on a chair. Feel for the sensation that you are seated more on the fronts of the sitting bones, and less rocking back into the flesh of the buttocks. This will help to maintain the natural curve of the low back and keep your spine as tall as possible.

Bring the tip of your fingers to the tip of your shoulders with your elbows wide, so your bent arms are like wings. As you exhale, bring your elbows together in front of your chest. As you inhale, bring your elbows up and then back. Follow the natural pattern of your breath and continue this fluid, circular movement. Take several cycles of breath in this sequence and then reverse directions for several cycles of breath. Take a few complete cycles of breath to rest and receive the energetic release.

Extending and flexing the spine to soothe the nervous system and move energy

Sit in a comfortable position on the ground or on a chair. Interlace your fingers at the back of your head. Allow the thumbs to extend down the sides of the neck and press the meat of your palms into the sides of your skull. Open the elbows comfortably away from each other and feel your hands lifting the weight of your skull off of your neck. As you inhale, lift your sternum toward the sky and raise your chin slightly away from your chest.

As you exhale, round your back body, lower your chin toward your chest and exhale through the mouth pressing the breath out, as though you could completely empty the body with your exhalation, drawing the belly button to the spine as you do so. Make some sound if you'd like, or use a lion's breath, exhaling with the mouth wide open and a roaring sound. With the back body rounded, go into your shell and breathe. This is tortoise energy. You are free to go into your shell at any time. Imagine that you are shielding yourself from anything that could harm you and anything that no longer serves you. Allow

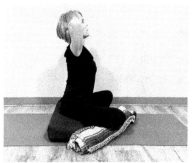 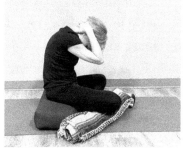

the past to be behind you. Consciously move out the energy of whatever you are letting go and putting to rest.

As you inhale deeply, open your throat and chest and draw the breath in fully. Lift your face, your chest, your rib cage, and draw into your being whatever you are consciously bringing into your life today. Repeat this sequence for a minute or longer. Fully integrate into every breath and every cell of your being your intention and resolve to leave behind what no longer serves you and to receive what is most beneficial for your wholeness, wellness, health, and vitality.

Twisting and lateral flexion, solo or as partners

If you are working with a group, you may choose to do this seated series as partner poses or solo. Begin seated in a comfortable position on the floor or on a chair. If you are working with a partner, come back to back with your partner. Each person extends the arms out to the side. If you are working with a partner, bring the back of your hands to touch the back of your partner's hands. Inhale to bring your arms overhead. Exhale to twist to the right, placing your left hand on your own right knee. If you are working with a partner, bring your own right hand to your partner's left knee.

If you are working solo, bring the right hand behind you. Inhaling, come to the center with arms extended over head. Exhaling, twist the other way, placing your right hand on your own left knee and extending your left hand behind you.

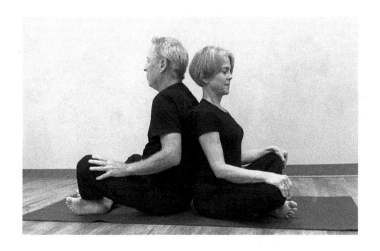

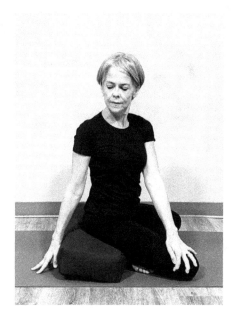

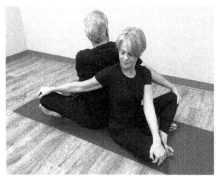
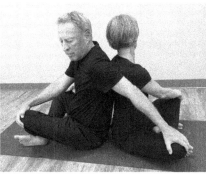

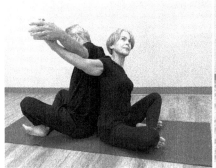
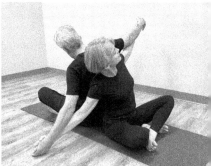

"If they ask you how rich you are,
tell them to look inside your heart."
~ **Matshona Dhliwayo**

If you are working with a partner, bring the left hand to your partner's right knee. Repeat this sequence multiple times, right and left.

After twisting several times to the right and to the left, inhale to come up center and bend laterally to one side and then to the other, moving on the breath, multiple times in each direction. If you are working back to back with a partner, explore the possibility of silently agreeing how to move together.

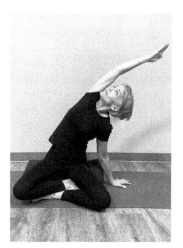
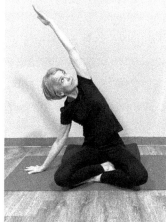

Mudra and meditation

A *mudra* is a seal or gesture, and another way to focus our attention and work with the subtle energy of the body. To practice *mudra* with the hands, sit calmly and quietly. If you are comfortable closing your eyes, this increases

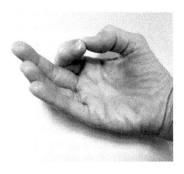

the healing power of the *mudra*, helping to maintain focus to witness the sensations that arise. The first step of *mudra* practice is to rub your hands together for 20 to 30 seconds to get the circulation going. You will feel warmth rising out of your hands from the friction, indicating activation of all the nerve endings in the hands, stimulating each cell linked to various organs. Next, place your hands onto your lap with palms facing up; quiet your thoughts to feel the tingling or pulsating sensations in your hands and your body. Stay in this position for about 15 seconds.

Jnana mudra, the seal of knowledge

After preparing the hands for *mudra* practice, bring the tip of the index finger of each hand to meet the tip of its corresponding thumb. Actively press the thumb and index finger one into the other, but be gentle; less is more. In this *mudra*, the thumbs represent universal consciousness – something 'higher' or greater than ourselves. The index fingers represent our individual consciousness – our mind and thoughts that create our own reality. By connecting the thumbs and forefingers we unite these two elements – the Self and the universe. The other three fingers of the hand extend actively away together. The circle we make with the index finger and thumb creates a 'seal' or '*pranic* circuit' so that the energy of our practice and meditation flows back into the body rather than 'leaking' from the ends of the fingertips. The simplest interpretation of *jnana mudra* is represented by the "zero" formed by the thumb and index finger: **"I know this much."**

Rest the back of the hands onto the thighs with the palms facing upwards. *Jnana mudra* is practiced with the palm facing upwards in a gesture of receptivity. *Chin mudra* employs a similar position of the fingers, but is performed with the palms facing downward. It is often confused with *jnana mudra* as they look so similar, but the direction of the palms downward is a more introspective gesture and said to have a grounding effect, encouraging our attention and focus to move inwards.

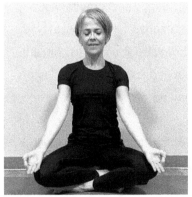 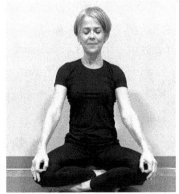

Supta badha konasana/reclined bound angle pose
This may activate and balance all of the chakras.

Ideally this pose is performed with several props – one or more blocks, a bolster, a blanket, and possibly a yoga strap. Set up your space by placing the block the medium height and ramping your bolster on the block. Place a folded blanket at the end of the bolster where your head will be. If you do not have access to these props, you can practice this posture on the ground with support for the head.

Once you have your props arranged, sit at the end of your bolster with the soles of your feet together. Use your own good judgment to decide how close to bring your heels toward your pelvis. Pain and discomfort in the hips and knees are your body's way of asking for more space and gentleness.

Open your feet like a book, and open to your story. You are so much more than your story, though you do bring your whole life, your whole story to this practice. Slide your shoulders blades to your back, down toward the waist. Lift your sternum to lengthen all sides of your spine. Rest your hands or forearms on your inner thighs and simultaneously press your thighs up into your hands or forearms as you press your hands or forearms down into your thighs. You are creating an isometric contraction, engaging the muscles of the inner thigh. Hold this action and breathe for five to ten deep, rhythmic breaths.

Release the contraction of the inner thigh muscles and relax the legs. Recline on your bolster, and adjust your props to

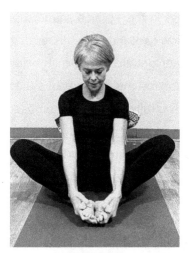

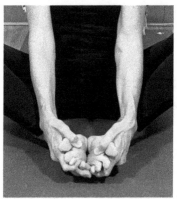

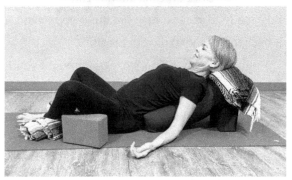

support your legs in this position and to support your spine, especially your low back and neck. This restorative posture is to open the body, not to stretch it. Stretching activates the nervous system. Relaxation restores the nervous system. Be sure every part of your body is fully supported by props so you truly relax. Honor the feedback from your body. Allow yourself to be in a physical posture that is truly comfortable.

Breathe here for several minutes. Feel the breath in the back of your body, on the backside of the energetic center of the heart. Using your breath as your anchor, allow yourself to dissolve into this pose. If this posture is not sustainable, or if you find it difficult to breathe deeply, adjust to a position that supports your breath and experience of relaxation.

Practice witness consciousness. See yourself, in this moment, responding to the breath moving in and out of the body, freely, easily. You do not need to work to manipulate or control the breath. Your body wants to breathe. Inhale through the nose into the throat, the chest, and the belly. As you exhale, lift the pelvic floor to the navel and draw the navel toward the spine. Once an exhalation is complete, your body rebounds, ready to receive new breath. If your mind strays, bring it back to the sound of your breath.

Honor your story. Your story has brought you to this moment, here and now. Your story is sacred, your life is sacred, and your mat is your sacred space. After a few moments, mindfully release the pose, roll to one side, and come to an upright position.

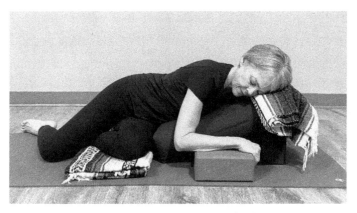

Supported spinal twist – twisting toward the earth

This twist uses a similar set of props as the supported *supta bada konasana*. Place a yoga block on the floor at medium height. Rest a bolster on the block and a blanket at the base of the bolster. Have a couple of additional blankets ready to use as arm rests and to cover yourself once you recline. Bring the dimple of the right hip against the bolster and fan your legs comfortably. Place your hands on either side of the bolster and round your back like a Halloween cat. Spin your belly button toward the bolster and recline forward. Bring one ear to the bolster, allowing the placement of the head to be a therapeutic position for your neck. Stay in this position and breathe for four or five minutes.

The healing methods of yoga use twists to release old energy. The yogis believe that grief and sadness is released through the back body. We distill and cleanse our energetic body as we twist toward the ground, yielding the weight of the physical and energetic body to the support of the stable, reliable earth. After four or five minutes, introduce just enough movement into the physical body to switch sides. Each new side is a new event. Adjust your props as necessary to rest comfortably in the twist. Once you have made all necessary adjustments, rest in stillness.

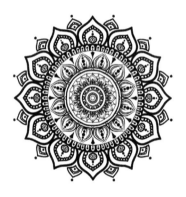

"Breath is the bridge which connects
life to consciousness,
which unites your body to your thoughts.
Whenever your mind becomes scattered,
use your breath as the means to
take hold of your mind again."
~ Thich Nhat Hanh

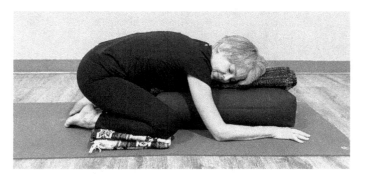

Balasana/child's pose – supported

Have you ever noticed how instinctively little children advocate for their own needs? And even very young infants learn the ability to comfort themselves in uncomfortable situations. Can you acknowledge and honor your own needs? Having needs does not make you needy; it makes you human.

Honor your body's wisdom and intelligence. Invite the thinking, analytical mind to take a break, and use your breath to move into the realm of feeling. Notice any tension in the physical body. Notice any inclination to stifle emotional releases. Rest when you need rest, and let go when you have an opportunity to let go – when the environment feels safe and supportive. What we don't express, we may repress, and this can lead to chronic holding patterns in the body, creating tension, pain, and even illness. The mind can lie, but the body cannot.

You are your own best authority on your body. A good teacher or doctor can bring expertise to point you in the direction of good choices to support your health and well-being. And the choices are yours to make.

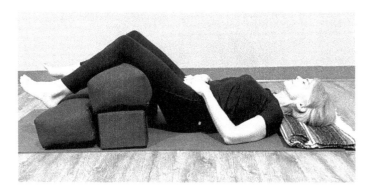

Savasana/final resting pose

We conclude every yoga practice with a still posture of deep restoration and renewal, so we return to *savasana*. The Sanskrit name of this posture comes from two words: *sava*, meaning "corpse," and *asana*, meaning "seat," or "pose." The practice of *savasana* invites us to take the posture of a corpse, resting completely motionless, with a still and quiet mind. *Savasana* offers a depth of release that goes beyond simple relaxation to a place deep and complete rest. Though it may appear to be an easy pose, *savasana* can require practice and experience. It is a posture of absolute surrender. Be patient with yourself if at first you find it difficult to rest like a corpse.

We work very hard in our lives, and many of us rarely take time to deeply rest. The practice of deep rest and relaxation manipulates the nervous system to a parasympathetic dominant state, resulting in measurable benefits such as:

>> the reduction of blood pressure
>> the lowering of serum triglycerides and blood sugar levels in the blood

- » an increase in "good cholesterol" levels
- » improvements in digestion, elimination, and fertility
- » and reduction of muscle tension, insomnia, and generalized fatigue

If you do no other yoga practice regularly, consider introducing a 15-20 minute *savasana* into your daily routine.

Lie on your back on a flat surface. Place a thin cushion or blanket under your head and neck, shaping the cushion so that it supports the natural curve in the neck. Let the arms rest away from the sides of the body and the legs rest apart from each other, arranging the four limbs equidistant from the spine and symmetrically on the ground. Adjust the arms until the shoulders relax, and adjust the legs until the low back and hips relax. For more comfort in the low back, place a cushion or bolster under the knees so that the low back, hips, and knees are all in some degree of flexion. Adjust the height of the prop to your optimal comfort. Mimicking the safety of our mother's womb, we bring every joint and the whole spine into flexion to quiet the nervous system. Also, symmetry in the physical body is gentle for the muscle of the heart and soothing to the mind. Attention to the alignment of your resting posture will make it more comfortable and relaxing.

As the body and mind sink into deeper states of relaxation, the core body temperature may drop, so cover yourself with a blanket. Adjust your props, your body, and your clothing, asking yourself the question, "Is there anything

I can do to make my position five-to-ten percent more comfortable?" When you are ready, close your eyes. Soften all the muscles of the face, especially the muscles around the sensory organs. You might cover your eyes with a small pillow.

Stages of *savasana*

There are various stages of *savasana*, though we may not experience all of them every time we practice the posture. The first stage is physiological relaxation. This includes physical, mental, and emotional relaxation. It may take at least 15 minutes to achieve complete relaxation. Thoughtful attention to the setup of the posture will support this.

In this first stage of *savasana*, like other restorative yoga postures and relaxation practices, you may experience waves of emotions and emotional release. If emotions well up to a point of discomfort, you might consider a side-lying *savasana* in a more fetal-like position as an alternative to lying on your back. A side-lying *savasana* could be naturally soothing and comforting. And even though there is no "prescribed" breath pattern for *savasana*, a deliberate pattern of breathing with exhalations that are longer than inhalations can quiet the mind and calm the nervous system. As one example, try inhaling deeply for about four counts, you might pause the breath for one or two counts, and then exhale for about six counts, until you feel like the exhalation is truly complete.

Consciousness exists all the time, but thoughts come and go. Unlike active, moving, and physically demanding poses, *savasana* requires a conscious decision to release the activity of the mind and surrender fully into a state of presence. The breath is like the wind shaping the mind in the way that the wind in nature shapes the oceans and the trees. If the mind is busy with many thoughts, engage the breath as an anchor to stay grounded in the present moment.

The second stage of *savasana* is *pratyahara*, a Sanskrit word that is usually translated as "sense withdrawal," but it can also be understood as "the introversion of the senses." This is the fifth of the eight limbs of yoga practice as described by Patanjali. In a state of *pratyahara*, our five senses are introverted and we lose ambition and curiosity about external stimuli.

The final stage of *savasana* is *ashunya*, a Sanskrit word meaning "non-emptiness." This is a state that we may not experience every time we practice *savasana*. We can only know the state of *ashunya* once we've "come back" from it. In the experience of *ashunya*, we are not sleeping or dreaming, but we go "somewhere else." Like the very high state of consciousness known as *samadhi*, in *ashunya*, there is no separation between the ego and the true Self. There is no "I"; only peacefulness and feelings of oneness with Source, or the universe. It is a blissful experience of pure, light, present being. *Ashunya* is not a state to be "sought after," but we might experience it when we create the space to do the work of relaxing completely and surrendering fully.

Coming out of *savasana*

After you have rested for several minutes – 20 minutes or even longer is ideal – be mindful of the way you come out of *savasana*. The more deeply relaxed you have been, the more carefully you must return to wakeful awareness of the external world.

One at a time, draw the knees to the chest. Slowly roll to one side and rest in the fetal position for several cycles of breath. You might open your eye while you're lying on your side, or wait until after you have gently made your way up to an easy seated position.

"Solitude is for me a fount of healing
which makes my life worth living."
~ Carl Jung

Guided grief visualization

This guided grief visualization may be considered an "advanced" practice, and is not necessarily recommended for someone who is in the early, raw stages of grief. Individual discernment in this practice is recommended. If you choose to experiment with this exercise or are leading this practice with a group, please give yourself or the group participants permission to practice total self-care. If at any time during the practice you or the participants need to pause, quit, or leave the room, please allow freedom to do so.

This exercise is an opportunity for you to be with your experience of grief in a different way. You are invited to take a journey that may allow you to understand and experience grief in a new way. This journey is just for you, and you can control it. The words for this visualized journey are words that I have chosen. Feel free to change them to better suit your own experience or needs.

If you would like to do this exercise, find a comfortable reclined or seated position. Adjust your props, your body, and your clothing so that you are completely comfortable. Close your eyes, and take a few deep breaths, inhaling through the nose and exhaling out through an open mouth, even creating a sighing sound as you exhale. Release the weight of the body and mind. Release tension and fatigue. As you breathe in, fill your body with peace and serenity. As you exhale, surrender your worries and fears.

Now breathe naturally, in and out through the nose, if possible, and bring your awareness to the sensations of the breath. Notice the movement and warmth of the breath on the skin beneath the nostrils. Notice how the shape of the body naturally changes as you receive and surrender the breath. You don't need to will it; the breath comes and goes as grace. There is no need to breathe in any specific way; simply let your breath serve as a tool to bring you to state of relaxed awareness, attentive without tension.

Without bias or judgment, notice your feelings. Notice the sensations of emotion that may be present. Name and acknowledge your feelings without identification or attachment. Feel them, acknowledge them, and let them be.

If you are comfortable, allow yourself to sink more deeply into a sense of safety and reassurance. Bring your awareness to the point between the eyebrows, in the mid-brain, just above the soft palate of the mouth. You might imagine a movie screen in your brain. Let this place come alive with your visualization.

In your mind's eye, visualize a place that is special for you, a place where you feel safe, secure, at ease, calm, happy, peaceful, content. This could be a room inside, or a place outside, a favorite park, lake, or vacation place. Maybe one place emerges in your mind immediately. Maybe you need a moment to choose. Take your time choosing your special place.

With your full awareness, let yourself really be "there." Notice as much sensory detail as possible.

❀ Notice everything you see. Notice all the colors around you, and the shape, texture, and form of various objects. Allow the image to become vivid in your mind.

❀ Notice everything you can hear: what sounds are present?

❀ Notice anything that you can feel: notice warmth and coolness, sensations on your skin, and anything you can touch.

❀ Notice everything you can smell: what scents and fragrances characterize this place?

❀ Notice anything that you can taste.

You might sit in your favorite place, or stand, or walk about, or lie down. Notice the bodily sensations and energetic experiences of your posture and movement. Notice how you feel in this place. Do you feel safe and at ease? Happy and energized? Quiet and contemplative? The a moment to fully notice your mind, your body, and your being in this special place.

In the distance, visualize a cloud or a mist. Notice that it appears to be moving toward you. As the mist comes closer, it begins to take the shape and form of your loved one who has died. As your loved one draws nearer, notice how he or she looks. Does your loved one approach quickly or slowly?

Notice how you are feeling? Excited? Frightened? Uncertain? Comforted?

Once your loved one is near enough, look at his or her face. What is the expression? Does he or she appear to be happy, calm, sad, or agitated? Look into his or her eyes.

Pause and notice your own feelings as you make eye contact with your loved one.

As you face your loved one, you have an opportunity to speak. There may be something that you didn't have an opportunity to say before, something important that you want to repeat, or something new that you want to share now. Take a moment, and allow the thought and statement to arise within you. Now imagine speaking to your loved one. Take some time here.

Now, it is your chance to hear your loved one speak to you. Listen as your loved one tells you somethings important. What does he or she have to say to you? Pause, listen, and notice how you feel.

Soon, it will be time for this particular encounter to end and for you to take leave of your loved one for now. Before you part company, ask your loved one for a gift that you can carry with you. The gift might be a few words, or a symbol or token of remembrance. What does your loved one give to you?

You might choose to give a parting gift to your loved one. What do you choose to give?

Now your loved one begins to move away from you. As the image becomes blurry and your loved one leaves your sight, breathe deeply and know that you can return to your special place any time to visit with your loved one, or just to feel safe, peaceful, and serene.

As you leave your special place, deepen your breath. Begin to notice your mind, your emotions, your feelings, and drop your awareness into your physical body. Listen to the sounds of the room in which you're resting and gradually extend your awareness into the environment of the room. Stretch your arms and legs, and blink your eyes open, allowing them to adjust to the light. Rest in silence for at least a moment or two. If you have practiced this exercise with a group, you may wish to share your experiences with the group after a suitable period of restful silence.

"All shall be well,
and all shall be well,
and all manner of things
shall be well."
~ Julian of Norwich

233

Sankalpa: resolve or intention

Establishing our heartfelt intention and creating a personal statement of that intention, or *sankalpa*, can be a powerful method for directing this transformational process and expending the energy of our life with purpose. Discovering a *sankalpa* is a process of self-study and listening to the heart. Establishing *sankalpa* is a spiritual practice. Often, the biggest mistake we make in spiritual practice is creating the belief that we need to be different than who we truly are. Our heartfelt desire is already present, waiting to be seen, heard, and felt. It's not something we need to make up, and the mind doesn't have to go wildly searching for it.

In addition to the questions suggested in the *svadhyaya* portion of this book, other questions for this self-study and heartfelt listening might include:

- *For what am I grateful?*
- *What are my gifts?*
- *What do I love?*
- *Who am I becoming?*
- *How can I serve?*
- *What is my inner knowing telling me about my life right now?*
- *If today were my last day, what would my intention be?*

It takes real courage to listen to the heart. A quiet, settled mind, cultivated through yoga and meditation, will best be able to hear the still, small voice within and welcome its message. When you hear the call, pause, create space, sit with it, feel it, and reflect on it.

A *sankalpa* statement is most powerful when expressed positively in the present tense. For example, rather than saying "I want to be happier and more open to life," try "I am happy and open to all that life brings me." Stating a *sankalpa* in present tense is an acknowledgment that whatever we desire most is already alive within us. We increase the power of a *sankalpa* statement by beginning with the words "I am grateful." Using this same example, an even stronger *sankalpa* would be "I am grateful to be happy and open to all that life brings me."

Establishing *sankalpa* empowers and liberates the yoga practitioner to take effective action. What action does your heartfelt desire require?

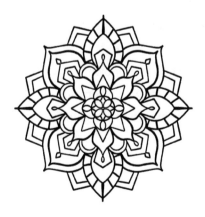

You are Free

Experiences of grief, transition, and loss can leave us feeling powerless. When events occur in our lives that were not of our choosing, it's good to remember that we are free to choose how we will navigate life after an experience of loss. Holidays, anniversaries, birthdays, and special occasions can be especially difficult after a loss. Anticipation of the event can sometimes be worse than the actual experience of it. Remember, you are free to choose if or how you will participate in any and all social festivities. There are no rules.

You are free to make your own decisions.

You are free to anticipate and plan ahead for holidays, anniversaries, and milestone moments.

You are free to choose to do something completely different than you've ever done before or than anyone in your family or circle of friends is choosing to do.

You are free to decide to not celebrate a holiday or occasion.

You are free to leave town or to stay home.

You are free to choose your own life-giving activities.

You are free to decide with whom you will spend time.

You are free to leave a party or gathering when you feel the need.

You are free to experience your emotions, without judging them or attaching to them or identifying with them.

You are free to cry.

You are free to cry in public.

You are free to include a deceased loved one in your holiday rituals by hanging his or her stocking, lighting a candle, preparing and enjoying a favorite food of the deceased, and sharing stories.

You are free to reminisce about the person who died.

You are free to laugh and have fun without guilt.

You are free to do something for others, even if you are hurting.

You are free to change your mind anytime.

You are free to be kind to yourself and practice self-care.

You are free to make your yoga practice part of your self-care plan, to put on your own oxygen mask first before assisting others, to get up every day, make a self-care plan for the day, and keep it.

"Be willing to be a beginner
every single morning."
~ Meister Eckhart

Create a practice that is sustainable for yourself over time

Life is like a river. It keeps on flowing, and as it does, it carves out the earth around it. Anything that appears to be solid is vulnerable to its current. Even when the river seems to be calm and still, it is in motion, creating change beneath its surface in ways we cannot know. Practicing *Yoga for Grief, Transition, and Loss* can help us do our best to remain fluid and flexible enough to adapt to new challenges, and at the same time firm, steady, and connected to reliable ground.

Find a rhythm for your practice that includes yoga breaks in the day, in the week, and over the course of a year. How much and how often will you practice? Show up for your own sake. Make daily, weekly, seasonal, and annual dates with yourself to do your practice. The practice is not so much a retreat from life, though sometimes we may simply need a break from the heaviness of grief. The practice becomes a means of transforming life. Practicing for even a few minutes each day helps to maintain consistent effort, devotion, and intention to be compassionate toward ourselves and others. Prioritizing practice creates a rhythm that supports self-compassion practice and a sense of flow in life.

Grief work is not passive. With effort, practice, patience, and support, we can survive grief and find integration around loss. *Yoga for Grief, Transition, and Loss* offers techniques for living in awareness of the present moment, making choices to direct the energy and flow of our life, taking effective action to care for ourselves and others, creating a rhythm of life and practice that is nourishing, and offering us a glimpse and a lived experience of our connection with Spirit.

A New You

Practicing *Yoga for Grief, Transition, and Loss* with purpose and intention is a transformational process. We will be changed, and we will not be able to fit our renewed being into old boxes. Self-limiting beliefs, ideas, and habits will fall away to create space for healthier and more nourishing ways of thinking, believing, and living. As we choose to face experiences and emotions that are unfamiliar, complicated, or difficult, we cultivate the habit of opening ourselves up for the sake of our personal integration and our connection with Spirit. I would not be the person I am today had I not experienced grief and loss, and I am grateful for who I am and for all that I am becoming.

"We're all just walking each other home."
~ Ram Dass

About the Author

*M*oya McGinn Mathews, E-RYT 500, YACEP®, was introduced to the practice of yoga in 2000, soon after the sudden death of her husband, Chad. The yoga class was held in the smelly basement of her gym, the teacher was authentic and she, the student, was willing. While standing on her mat in Warrior 2, arms stretched wide open, heart exposed and vulnerable, she thought to herself, "I don't know what this is, but I know I need to do it."

Since that day, she has logged thousands of hours of study and teaching experience with students of every level, from absolute beginners to advanced teacher trainees, students of every age, from five to 85+, students in various stages of life working with special circumstances and conditions, from pregnant to postpartum moms, students with arthritis or other conditions of chronic pain, students suffering with anxiety or depression, and students navigating grief and loss.

Her formal academic work includes a Bachelor of Arts in Music from the College of St. Benedict in St. Joseph, MN, and graduate studies in Theology and Ministry at the St. Paul Seminary School of Divinity of the University of St. Thomas in St. Paul, MN. She has worked in parish ministry for more than 40 years and has supported hundreds of bereaved people on the journey of grief and loss.

Printed in the USA
CPSIA information can be obtained
at www.ICGtesting.com
JSHW010111231123
52628JS00012B/187